Robotic Technologies in Biomedical and Healthcare Engineering

Biomedical and Robotics Healthcare

Series Editors:
Utku Kose, Jude Hemanth, Omer Deperlioglu

Robotic Technologies in Biomedical and Healthcare Engineering
Deepak Gupta, Moolchand Sharma, Vikas Chaudhary and Ashish Khanna

Artificial Intelligence for the Internet of Health Things
Deepak Gupta, Eswaran Perumal and K. Shankar

Mechano-Electric Correlations in the Human Physiological System
A. Bakiya, K. Kamalanand and R. L. J. De Britto

Biomedical Signal and Image Examination with Entropy-Based Techniques
V. Rajinikanth, K. Kamalanand, C. Emmanuel and B. Thayumanavan

For more information about this series, please visit: https://www.routledge.com/ Biomedical-and-Robotics-Healthcare/book-series/BRHC

Robotic Technologies in Biomedical and Healthcare Engineering

Edited by
Deepak Gupta, Moolchand Sharma,
Vikas Chaudhary, and Ashish Khanna

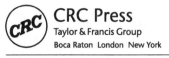

CRC Press
Taylor & Francis Group
Boca Raton London New York

CRC Press is an imprint of the
Taylor & Francis Group, an **informa** business

First edition published 2021
by CRC Press
6000 Broken Sound Parkway NW, Suite 300, Boca Raton, FL 33487-2742

and by CRC Press
2 Park Square, Milton Park, Abingdon, Oxon, OX14 4RN

© 2021 Taylor & Francis Group, LLC

CRC Press is an imprint of Taylor & Francis Group, LLC

Library of Congress Cataloging-in-Publication Data
Names: Gupta, Deepak, editor. | Sharma, Moolchand, editor. | Chaudhary,
Vikas, editor. | Khanna, Ashish, editor.
Title: Robotic technologies in biomedical and healthcare engineering /
edited by Deepak Gupta, Moolchand Sharma, Vikas Chaudhary, Ashish Khanna.
Description: First edition. | Boca Raton : CRC Press, 2021. | Series:
Biomedical and robotics healthcare | Includes bibliographical references
and index. | Summary: "This book aims at exhibiting the latest research
achievements, findings, and ideas in the field of robotics in biomedical
and healthcare engineering, primarily focusing on the walking assistive
robot, telerobotic surgery, upper/lower limb rehabilitation, and
radiosurgery, etc"—Provided by publisher.
Identifiers: LCCN 2021000626 (print) | LCCN 2021000627 (ebook) |
ISBN 9780367624187 (hardback) | ISBN 9781003112273 (ebook)
Subjects: LCSH: Biomedical engineering. | Medical care—Technological
innovations. | Robots.
Classification: LCC R856 .R63 2021 (print) | LCC R856 (ebook) |
DDC 610.28—dc23
LC record available at https://lccn.loc.gov/2021000626
LC ebook record available at https://lccn.loc.gov/2021000627

ISBN: 978-0-367-62418-7 (hbk)
ISBN: 978-0-367-63133-8 (pbk)
ISBN: 978-1-003-11227-3 (ebk)

Typeset in Times
by codeMantra

Dr. Deepak Gupta would like to dedicate this book to his father Sh. R. K. Gupta, his mother Smt. Geeta Gupta for their constant encouragement, his family members including his wife, brothers, sisters, and kids, and his students close to his heart.

Mr. Moolchand Sharma would like to dedicate this book to his father Sh. Naresh Kumar Sharma and his mother Smt. Rambati Sharma for their constant support and motivation, and his family members including his wife Ms. Pratibha Sharma and Son Dhairya Sharma. He would also like to give his special thanks to the publisher and other co-editors for having faith in his abilities. Before all and after all, he thanks the Almighty God.

Dr. Vikas Chaudhary would like to dedicate this book to his father, Sh. Rajendra Singh, his mother Smt. Santosh for their constant support and motivation, and his family members including his wife Ms. Amita Panwar, his daughter Astha Chaudhary, and Sons Shivansh Chaudhary and Anmol Chaudhary. He would also like to give his special thanks to the publisher and other co-editors for having faith in his abilities. Before all and after all, he thanks the Almighty God.

Dr. Ashish Khanna dedicates this book to his (late) father Shree RC Khanna and his mother Smt. Surekha Khanna and his family.

Contents

Preface

We hereby are delighted to launch our book entitled *Robotic Technologies in Biomedical and Healthcare Engineering.* The rapid progress of the Robotic and Artificial Intelligence technique provides new opportunities for biomedical and healthcare engineering. Today's modern world is currently under a significant influence on innovative technologies such as Artificial Intelligence, Deep Learning, Robotics, and IoT. This book aims to present the various approaches, techniques, and their applications that are available in the field of biomedical and healthcare. It is a valuable source of knowledge for researchers, engineers, practitioners, and graduate and doctoral students working in the same field. It will also be useful for faculty members of graduate schools and universities. Around 30 full-length chapters have been received. Among these manuscripts, nine chapters have been included in this volume. All the chapters submitted were peer-reviewed by at least two independent reviewers, who were provided with a detailed review pro forma. The comments from the reviewers were communicated to the authors, who incorporated the suggestions in their revised manuscripts. The recommendations from two reviewers were taken into consideration while selecting chapters for inclusion in the volume. The exhaustiveness of the review process is evident, given the large number of articles received addressing a wide range of research areas. The stringent review process ensured that each published chapter met the rigorous academic and scientific standards.

We would also like to thank the authors of the published chapters for adhering to the time schedule and for incorporating the review comments. We wish to extend our heartfelt acknowledgment to the authors, peer-reviewers, committee members, and production staff whose diligent work put shape to this volume. We especially want to thank our dedicated team of peer-reviewers who volunteered for the arduous and tedious step of quality checking and critique on the submitted chapters.

Deepak Gupta,
Moolchand Sharma,
Vikas Chaudhary,
Ashish Khanna

Editors

Deepak Gupta is an eminent academician and plays versatile roles and responsibilities juggling between lectures, research, publications, consultancy, community service, Ph.D. and post-doctorate supervision, and so on. With 13 years of rich expertise in teaching and two years in the industry, he focuses on rational and practical learning. He has contributed massive literature in the fields of Human–Computer Interaction, Intelligent Data Analysis, Nature-Inspired Computing, Machine Learning, and Soft Computing. He is working as an Assistant Professor at the Maharaja Agrasen Institute of Technology (GGSIPU), Delhi, India. He has served as Editor-in-Chief, Guest Editor, and Associate Editor in SCI and various other reputed journals (Elsevier, Springer, Wiley, and MDPI). He has actively been part of various reputed international conferences. He is not only backed with a strong profile, but his innovative ideas, research end-results, and the notion of implementation of technology in the medical field are by and large contributing to the society significantly. He is currently a Post-Doc researcher at the University of Valladolid, Spain. He has completed his first Post-Doc from Inatel, Brazil, and Ph.D. from Dr. APJ Abdul Kalam Technical University. He has authored/edited 47 books with national-/international-level publishers (Elsevier, Springer, Wiley, and Katson). He has published 162 scientific research publications in reputed international journals and conferences including 83 SCI Indexed Journals of IEEE, Elsevier, Springer, Wiley, and many more. He has also filed three patents. He is the Editor-in-Chief of OA Journal-Computers and Quantum Computing and Applications (QCAA); Associate Editor of Expert Systems (Wiley), Intelligent Decision Technologies (IOS Press), and Journal of Computational and Theoretical Nanoscience; and Honorary Editor of ICSES Transactions on Image Processing and Pattern Recognition. He is also a series editor of "Elsevier Biomedical Engineering" (Elsevier), "Intelligent Biomedical Data Analysis" (De Gruyter, Germany), "Explainable AI (XAI) for Engineering Applications" (CRC Press), and "Computational Intelligence for Data Analysis" (Bentham Science). He is appointed as Consulting Editor at Elsevier. He is also associated with various professional bodies like IEEE, ISTE, IAENG, IACSIT, SCIEI, ICSES, UACEE, Internet Society, SMEI, IAOP, and IAOIP and invited as a Faculty Resource Person/Session Chair/Reviewer/TPC member in different FDP, conferences, and journals. He is the convener of the 'ICICC' conference series.

Moolchand Sharma is currently an Assistant Professor in the Department of Computer Science and Engineering at the Maharaja Agrasen Institute of Technology, GGSIPU, Delhi. He has published scientific research publications in reputed international journals and conferences including SCI-indexed and Scopus-indexed journals such as Cognitive Systems Research (Elsevier), Physical Communication (Elsevier), Intelligent Decision Technologies: An International Journal, Cyber-Physical Systems (Taylor & Francis Group), International Journal of Image & Graphics

(World Scientific), International Journal of Innovative Computing and Applications (Inderscience), and Innovative Computing and Communication Journal (Scientific Peer-reviewed Journal). He has authored/co-authored chapters with international publishers like Elsevier, Wiley, and De Gruyter. He has also authored/edited three books with national-/international-level publishers (CRC Press and Bhavya publications). His research area includes Artificial Intelligence, Nature-Inspired Computing, Security in Cloud Computing, Machine Learning, and Search Engine Optimization. He is associated with various professional bodies like ISTE, IAENG, ICSES, UACEE, Internet Society, and so on. He possesses teaching experience of more than eight years. He is the co-convener of the ICICC-2018, ICICC-2019, and ICICC-2020 Springer conference series and also the co-convener of ICCRDA-2020 Scopus-Indexed IOP Materials Science & Engineering conference series. He is also a reviewer of many reputed journals from Springer, IEEE, Wiley, Taylor & Francis Group, and World Scientific Journal as well as of many Springer conferences. He is currently a doctoral researcher at the DCR University of Science & Technology, Haryana. He completed his Post Graduation in 2012 from SRM University, NCR Campus, Ghaziabad, and Graduation in 2010 from KNGD Modi Engg. College, GBTU.

Vikas Chaudhary is a Professor in the Computer Science & Engineering department at JIMS Engineering Management Technical Campus, Greater Noida. He has 18 years of teaching and research experience. He has obtained a Doctorate from the National Institute of Technology, Kurukshetra, India, in the field of Machine Learning/Unsupervised Learning. He has published various research papers in the International Journals of Springer, Elsevier, and Taylor & Francis. In addition, he has published various papers in IEEE International Conferences and national conferences. He is a reviewer of Springer Journal as well as of many IEEE conferences. He has written a book on Cryptography & Network Security. His research areas are Machine Learning and Artificial Neural Networks.

Dr. Ashish Khanna has expertise in Teaching, Entrepreneurship, and Research & Development with a specialization in Computer Science Engineering Subjects. He received his Ph.D. degree from the National Institute of Technology, Kurukshetra in March 2017. He has completed his M. Tech. and B. Tech. from GGSIPU, Delhi. He has completed his PDF from the Internet of Things Lab at Inatel, Brazil. He has around 136 accepted and published research papers and book chapters in reputed SCI, Scopus journals, conferences, and reputed book series including 61 papers in SCI-indexed Journals of IEEE Transaction, Springer, Elsevier, IEEE, and Wiley Journals. Additionally, he has authored and edited, and is editing 30 books for some of the top publishers like Springer, Wiley, Elsevier, and many more. He is a Series Editor in top publishing houses like Elsevier and De Gruyter (Germany) of the "Intelligent Biomedical Data Analysis" series. Furthermore, he has served in the research field as a Faculty Resource Person/Session Chair/Reviewer/TPC member in various conferences and journals. He has received the best paper award at a Springer international conference. He has also been invited as a Keynote Speaker. His research interests include Distributed Systems and their variants (MANET, FANET,

VANET, and IoT), Machine Learning, Evolutionary Computing, and many more. He is currently working at the Department of Computer Science and Engineering, Maharaja Agrasen Institute of Technology, under GGSIPU, Delhi, India. He is the convener and organizer of the ICICC-2018, 2019, and 2020 Springer conferences. He played a key role in the origination of a reputed publishing house "Bhavya Books" having 250 solution books and around 60 textbooks. He is also the originator of a research unit under the banner of "Universal Innovator". He has designed question papers for multiple government organizations. He has also played a key role in promoting Smart India Hackathon at MAIT. He also serves as a guest editor in various reputed international journals of Wiley, Inderscience, IGI Global, Bentham science, and many more. He is also currently editing some books of Elsevier, Springer, CRC Press, and Wiley, which will be published soon. His Cumulative Impact Factor (CIF) is around 180. He is a Series Editor in De Gruyter (Germany) of the "Intelligent Biomedical Data Analysis" series. His research interests include Image processing, Distributed Systems, and their variants (MANET, FANET, VANET, and IoT), Machine Learning, Evolutionary Computing, and many more.

List of Contributors

João André
Center for MicroElectroMechanical
  Systems,
University of Minho, Guimarães,
  Portugal

Panjavarnam Bose
Department of Electronics &
  Communication Engineering
Sri Sairam Engineering College
Chennai, Tamil Nadu, India

João Cerqueira
Clinical Academic Center (2CA-Braga)
Hospital of Braga
Braga, Portugal

Swati Goel
School of Computer and Systems
  Sciences
Jawaharlal Nehru University
New Delhi, India

T. Jayasankar
Electronics and Communication
  Engineering Department, University
  College of Engineering (BIT
  Campus)
Anna University
Tiruchirappalli, Tamil Nadu, India.

S. Jeelani
Oral Medicine and Radiology
Sri Venkateshwara Dental College
Ariyur, Puducherry, India

Kalpna Katiyar
Department of Biotechnology
Dr. Ambedkar Institute of Technology
  for Handicapped
Kanpur, Uttar Pradesh, India

S. Kirthikka
Department of Electronics &
  Communication Engineering
Sri Sairam Engineering College,
  Chennai, India

João M. Lopes
Center for MicroElectroMechanical
  Systems,
University of Minho, Guimarães,
  Portugal

Kajol Mohanty
Department of Electronics &
  Communication Engineering
Sri Sairam Engineering College
Chennai, Tamil Nadu, India

Preeti Nagrath
Department of Computer Science and
  Engineering
Bharati Vidyapeeth's College of
  Engineering
New Delhi, India

Manuel Palermo
Center for Microelectromechanical
  Systems
University of Minho
Guimarães, Portugal

António Pereira
Center for Microelectromechanical
  Systems
University of Minho
Guimarães, Portugal

Eswaran Perumal
Department of Computer Applications
Alagappa University
Karaikudi, Tamil Nadu, India

Denis A. Pustokhin
Department of Logistics
State University of Management
Moscow, Russia

Irina V. Pustokhina
Department of Entrepreneurship and
    Logistics
Plekhanov Russian University of
    Economics
Moscow, Russia

Rehab A. Rayan
Department of Epidemiology
High Institute of Public Health,
    Alexandria University
Qism Bab Sharqi, Egypt

Nuno Ribeiro
Center for Microelectromechanical
    Systems
University of Minho
Guimarães, Portugal

Cristina P. Santos
Center for Microelectromechanical
    Systems
University of Minho
Guimarães, Portugal

Eva Sarin
Department of Computer Science and
    Engineering
Bharati Vidyapeeth's College of
    Engineering
New Delhi, India

Mithileysh Sathiyanarayanan
Research & Innovation
MIT Square
Bangalore, India

Aparna Seth
Department of Biotechnology
Dr. Ambedkar Institute of Technology
    for Handicapped
Kanpur, Uttar Pradesh, India

K. Shankar
Department of Computer Applications
Alagappa University
Karaikudi, Tamil Nadu, India

Sumathi Sokkanarayanan
Department of Electronics &
    Communication Engineering
Sri Sairam Engineering College
Chennai, Tamil Nadu, India

Aditya Srivastava
Department of Biotechnology
Dr. Ambedkar Institute of Technology
    for Handicapped
Kanpur, Uttar Pradesh, India

S. Stephe
Electronics and Communication
    Engineering Department, University
    College of Engineering (BIT
    Campus)
Anna University
Tiruchirappalli, Tamilnadu, India

Subiksha S.
Department of Electronics &
    Communication Engineering
Sri Sairam Engineering College
Chennai, Tamil Nadu, India

Sujal B. H.
Department of Electronics &
    Communication Engineering
Sri Sairam Engineering College
Chennai, Tamil Nadu, India

Soham Taneja
Department of Computer Science and
  Engineering
Bharati Vidyapeeth's College of
  Engineering
New Delhi, India

Christos Tsagkaris
Faculty of Medicine
University of Crete
Heraklion, Greece

Vividha
Department of Computer Science and
  Engineering
Bharati Vidyapeeth's College of
  Engineering
New Delhi

Imran Zafar
Department of Bioinformatics and
  Computational Biology
Virtual University of Pakistan
Lahore, Pakistan

1 IoT-Integrated Robotics in the Health Sector

Rehab A. Rayan
Alexandria University

Christos Tsagkaris
University of Crete

Imran Zafar
Virtual University of Pakistan

CONTENTS

INTRODUCTION

Nowadays, the elderly population is growing worldwide with an increase in comorbidities due to their unhealthy modern habits like smoking, increased alcohol consumption, unhealthy diet, obesity, and the lack of physical activity. The World Health Organization (WHO) predicts that the health Internet of things (IoT) industry will explode, costing billions of dollars. Gradually, the IoT start-ups are introducing modern healthcare applications for integrating networked sensors to improve diagnosis, monitoring, and treatment of patients. Such applications are medical wearables for active monitoring of patient data or hospital networks and procedures, optimizing healthcare delivery and monitoring patient compliance (WHO 2013).

IoT is a promising option in the health sector, connecting applications, devices, and people to improve management of diseases with better outcomes and fewer errors, thus ensuring high efficiency and safe healthcare at lower costs (Patel et al. 2017). Integrating swiftly advancing technologies such as robotics, machine learning (ML), and the IoT could shift the way of living. Robotics involves machines programmed for labor-intensive jobs, while ML implies that computers and other devices operate with no prior programming. Integrating robotics and ML gives rise to robots that function independently. ML techniques range from supervised and semi-supervised learning to unsupervised learning, including pattern recognition statistically, parametric or non-parametric algorithms, neural networks, and other systems. ML coupled with the IoT could link many robots facilitating networking among individuals and things, sending data without intervening, and hence collecting and monitoring data within the network, for example, monitoring the environment, managing infrastructures, energy, and productions, and digitizing buildings, houses, transportation, and the health sector.

This chapter discusses the applications of adopting robotics and the IoT in the health sector. It explores the integration of robotics with the IoT for health applications, opportunities, and limitations, along with future insights.

HISTORY

The term "Robot", derived from the term "Robota", implying obligatory worker, was initially introduced in a play in 1921. The Robotics Institute of America defines a robot as a likewise human machine that is programmed to operate insensitively to the mechanical tasks of a human. In the 1940s, robots were regulated by three rules: causing no harm to humans, complying with human orders unless those breaching the first rule, and securing their own presence unless such security conflicts with the first or second rule. Robots were primarily designed to function similarly to man, and later, with added characteristics, they turned into smart machines.

HEALTH ROBOTICS

In the health sector, robots carry out coordinated tasks such as patient monitoring, clinical interventions, artificial prosthetics, rehabilitation, and e-health, applying electronics and mechanics such as measuring space, motion, or force, sensor technology, and others (Butter et al. 2008). Robotics could be valuable from the economic, social, and healthcare aspects where they could particularly benefit patient groups with special needs like amputees, stroke survivors, or those with mental insufficiencies. In the health sector, robotics could be applied in intelligent medical capsules, surgeries, prosthetics, analyzing and managing motor coordination, robot-aided social and cognitive treatment, and patient monitoring systems (Butter et al. 2008).

Lately, the medical robots' market is growing, and they are being used broadly worldwide in healthcare since they could evidently function timely at minimal risk, for example, in cardiac and prostatic operations, rehabilitation, and smart prosthetics. Social robotics could monitor and motivate patients (Martinez 2020). The exponential rise in innovative applications of robotics in the health sector is brought by the increasing need for information technology, which would derive future growth in the market. Globally, more application of the least invasive surgical robots is coupled with population growth, maintaining robustness in disorders like orthopedics, neurological disorders, and others. Adopting robotics is witnessed to be promising in countries such as China, India, and Brazil (Martinez 2020).

In today's surgical operations, computer-integrated systems perform more precisely than surgeons, especially in unfavorable settings where they provide technical solutions and smoothly monitor operations-needed data online added to operating on sensitive anatomical structures in dangerous proximity settings. Robotics, a multidisciplinary domain, linking the data in real world with the physical one, integrating engineering, computational science, biomechanics, sports science, biomedicine, neurology, cognitive science, and others, and hence coordinating sensors, motors, and humans, is challenging in various settings (Taylor 2006).

When using robotics in the health sector, the structure, movement, and intelligence, among other factors, should be considered. The structure describes the human engaging levels in supervising the functioning robots in typical procedures, especially when encountering system errors. The movement comprises programmed pathways for motion within the environment. Intelligence describes the inherent expert skill or knowledge facilitating carrying out jobs with minimal skill or knowledge than expected for a human doing the same job (Bakhru 2017).

APPLICATIONS OF ROBOTICS IN THE HEALTH SECTOR

In prevention, no treatment is required; however, for any detected abnormality, the diagnosis could be done by a robot (Butter et al. 2008). For instance, Toyota has designed the Balance Training Assist where a two-wheel robot displays games on the monitor using the data fed into the machine while the patient moves his/her weight (Toyota 2019). Using robots in surgeries would enable accuracy, reliability, and consistency acting on the human body especially in tiny spaces compared to physicians' performance, for instance, in microsurgery, minimally invasive surgery, nanobots, remote surgery via the IoT systems, robotics-assisted surgery, and other medical interventions. Nanobots, also called steerable surgeons, are applied in ocular disorders, for which they are manufactured with flat nickel elements and operated on magnetic fields using extrinsic electromagnetic coils (Tomlinson 2018).

Hospital robots for professional care are used for the aging population, for monitoring, assisting healthcare providers, providing physical activities, and other paramedic jobs (*The Journal of mHealth* 2018). For instance, Cody, a humanoid portable operator, applies direct physical interface (DPI) to help a healthcare provider in directly managing robot mobility, which in turn directly contacts the human body and responds to the patient's motion (Grifantini 2010).

Rehabilitation is provided in a healthcare facility or at home and includes sustaining muscle or motor coordination therapies. The behavior of patients is a key player in mental disorders. In the cerebral and nervous muscular system disorders, the brain functions inadequately and might cause disabilities in the lower extremities. Hybrid assistive limb, a cyborg-kind robot, could support and improve the wearer physically via supporting the lower extremities in movement based on the patient's needs (Ackerman 2018; Lazarte 2014). Robots can assist in everyday life activities such as performing those activities, supporting the movement for the disabled, and substituting organs via smart prosthetics. For example, Friend, the electrical wheelchair, is composed of a robotic arm, a computer, sensors, and joysticks to work on the system enabling the individual to read a book while turning pages (Souppouris 2012).

THE HEALTH IOT

The IoT can be vaguely defined as the Internet-based interconnection of computing devices embedded in everyday objects, enabling them to send and receive data. The IoT applications can be summarized with the following four principles: data collection, data conversion, data storage, and data processing. Interconnected devices including sensors, monitors, detectors, equators, and cameras collect data. Their input is converted from the analog form to the digital form enabling further processing. As data accumulate, storage is facilitated by means of cloud-based systems. At the end of the day, further data processing through advanced analytic modalities provides healthcare professionals with information necessary for decision-making (Psiha and Vlamos 2017; Latif et al. 2017; O'Brolcháin, de Colle, and Gordijn 2019). Although the human healthcare workforce can follow these principles as well, the IoT ensures the continuous flow of data facilitating instant decisions.

In the context of healthcare, IoT applications are expected to focus on research, clinical practice, and patient management, which are greatly discussed. Using the IoT in the healthcare system enables monitoring chronic diseases, care for elderly patients, and managing healthcare systems, among others. The IoT in the health sector could be service- or application-centered as shown in Figure 1.1. To the extent that insurance and industry intersect with healthcare, IoT applications in these fields may also impact healthcare (Mittelstadt 2017; Psiha and Vlamos 2017; Bandyopadhyay and Sen 2011; Gopal et al. 2019). When it comes to patients, the IoT infrastructure consists mostly of wearable devices. Wearables may include monitors for oxygen saturation, blood pressure, pulse/heart rate, and glucose level depending on the history of the patient and the parameters that should be monitored (Özdemir and Hekim 2018; Gopal et al. 2019; Gope and Hwang 2016). When it comes to physicians, the IoT offers real-time connection to their patients, to their colleagues, and to their clinic or laboratory. A cardiologist can be notified about an arrhythmia affecting one of his patients and a diabetologist can be informed about hypoglycemia threatening one of his patients. In both cases, the patients can have immediate medical guidance and support. At the same time, physicians can assess patients' adherence. It is not only a matter of outcome – e.g. blood pressure increases in case patients neglect their treatment – it can also be a matter of device monitoring. The delivery of this information to remote healthcare providers, such as a physician supervising a nursery home or a specialist consulting patient residing in remote communities, is also of great importance (Chai et al. 2019; Stefano and Kream 2018).

IOT-BASED ROBOTICS FRAMEWORK

The Internet would connect the robot's real and virtual world including the evolving robotic operating system (ROS), connectivity with the Bluetooth, and an application programming interface (API) as shown in Figure 1.2, where the robot would be a component of the IoT and could smoothly communicate with the cloud. Such robots are promising to have intelligent mobility and setting-oriented computing to the Internet relevant to the close physical ecosystem. The cloud would enable the robot to communicate either asynchronously or synchronously with any device, service, or business process on the cloud.

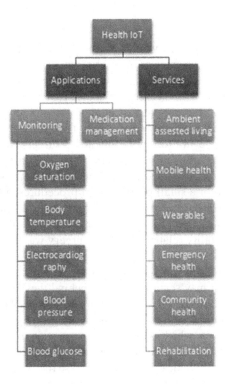

FIGURE 1.1   Health IoT.

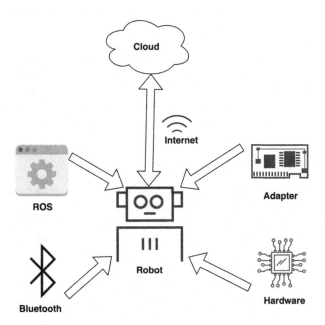

FIGURE 1.2   The IoT-based robotics framework.

DISCUSSION

Discussing healthcare robotics would resemble science fiction, if we could not discuss the real-world experience of integrating robots in healthcare. The da Vinci surgical robots as well as the nursing robots, which are currently being tested in Japan, provide sufficient grounds for such a discussion. According to a long-term study in Korea, the da Vinci robotic procedures were mainly performed in general surgery (~45%) and urologic surgery (~33%). To a smaller extent, the da Vinci procedures were applied in otorhinolaryngologic surgery, obstetric and gyneco-logic surgery, thoracic and cardiac surgery, and neurosurgery. The majority of surgeries (94.5%) were performed for malignancies, while surgeries for benign conditions accounted for a small portion of all procedures, although the numbers thereof have been steadily increasing. The study reported satisfactory results in terms of steadiness and safety. System malfunctions and failures were reported in 185 (1.8%) cases. Mortality related to robotic surgery was observed for 12 (0.12%) cases (Koh et al. 2018).

In Japan, about 5,000 nursing-care homes are testing robots for use in nursing care. As awkward as it may seem, the reason behind these figures is the declining number of human healthcare personnel in nursery homes. At the same time, 34.7 million are aged 65 and above, which equals more than a quarter of Japan's popula-tion. With this proportion, which is the highest proportion in these countries, getting only worse in the future as the population shrinks further by 2050, nursing robot sys-tems are expected to assist bedridden patients. These robots are typically confined to patient chambers. They can offer help with small services, such as fetching items or rearranging a patient's posture, carrying out laundry services and household chores, and even waking patients from sleep with a human-like voice. Nursing robots are also capable of administering. It has to be pointed out that although at the moment robots are supposed to administer any medical treatment to a patient, they could be programmed to do so (Grasso 2018). Compared to humans, nursing robots have a smaller learning curve, a lower operational cost, and are suitable for repetitive tasks. They can undertake not only time-consuming but also dangerous nursing duties, easing the occupational burden and exposure to hazardous infectious diseases or chemicals (Broadbent et al. 2016; Cao et al. 2017a).

OPPORTUNITIES AND CHALLENGES

Nowadays, relying on a robot surgeon is growing and gaining more acceptance in several specialties. Many hospitals are interested in the new generations of robotic surgical models that would solve both the functional and financial limitations of the existing robotic systems. Wintergreen Research has estimated that by 2021, the marketplace for robotic surgery would grow to approximately USD 20 billion. With the help of information technology, a robotic system might be capable physically to operate and interact automatically in both the real and virtual worlds. A robotic system could assimilate inputs from the real world, form a contextual sense, and then react based on both its programming and what it has newly gained. Such perception, control, and interaction insights yet lack sensibility (Patel et al. 2017).

Robotic systems, such as the da Vinci surgical robot, have already been in use worldwide during the past decade. The technical quality of the operations has increased, while the time of hospitalization and the post-operative need for rehabilitation have decreased. Other robotic systems are capable of sterilizing equipment, drawing blood, and monitoring patients' vitals (Dervaderics 2007; Koh et al. 2018). Robotic systems are also capable of supporting supply chains and logistics (Bedaf, Gelderblom, and De Witte 2015). Moreover, exoskeletons have been proven valuable for patients and healthcare workers, assisting paralyzed individuals to become more functional and non-paralyzed individuals to perform difficult or tiring tasks (Bogue 2009). The integration of this technology to healthcare facilities will raise the educational standards of health professionals (Özdemir and Hekim 2018). A higher level of digital literacy will empower physicians and allied professionals, and may pave new paths for research in terms of methods and interventions.

Robotic systems for patient monitoring and nursing homes can improve the healthcare workforce's resilience by performing regular, and in many cases monotonous, tasks or supporting debilitated patients' motility (Özdemir and Hekim 2018; Alaiad and Zhou 2014). Novel research focuses on the development of robotic behavioral architecture compatible with the needs of children or mentally debilitated individuals (Cao et al. 2017b). What is more, robots have favorable cost-effectiveness features. Hospital administrators have indicated that robots can lead to a 65% decrease in human labor cost yearly (Broadbent et al. 2016). Finally, yet importantly, robots can transcribe and store crucial medical information, minimizing the possibility of error as well as helping doctors and nurses to diagnose patients and even assisting lower-skilled health workers to administer treatment to patients with less input from doctors or other higher-skilled professionals (Challacombe 2013; Yoon and Lee 2019).

On the other hand, health robotics challenges should not be overlooked. In short, these challenges pertain to dependence on technology and dehumanization of healthcare. What will happen in case a robotic counter or a robotic sterilization system breaks down? Is the hospital going to postpone the delivery of medicines and supplies or the daily operations? Although this claim seems exaggerated now, it is something that we need to consider in the long run (Alaiad and Zhou 2014; Fracastoro et al. 2005). The dehumanization of healthcare has already been addressed in the context of the biomedical and biopsychosocial healthcare paradigms. There are fears that technology is linked to a feeling of superiority among healthcare providers resulting in a regression of healthcare to the paternalistic model of the previous centuries. This challenge becomes more complicated with robots in the field (Challacombe 2013). Monotonous everyday tasks, such as vitals monitoring, clinical examination, and phlebotomy, provide patients with an opportunity to communicate with their carers, build trust, and address their concerns. This is not the case for a robotic phlebotomist or exoskeleton though.

FUTURE INSIGHTS

Research reports that the future is IoT, hence the need for smooth development tools linking the physical world to IoT networks. The ROS could enable IoT platform-infrastructure connectivity where it holds a top level of abstraction for accessing hardware and could be integrated swiftly into the platform. However, not all these solutions are trustworthy (Hax et al. 2013). Lately, robotics has played a key role in medical operations, while researchers are attempting to reduce the ROS's electrome-chanical limitations using affordable and smaller devices, requiring fewer installing times via a skillful team that could be monitored distantly. However, adopting IoT in the health sector is booming, and there are some challenges involving advanced health monitoring technologies and costly medical devices among other aspects.

The rapidly growing healthcare at both clinic and home settings necessitates applying advanced remote sensors that could communicate with healthcare providers and caregivers and hence reaching the goal of IoT-integrated robotics. At the same time, tertiary/university hospitals can be an incubator for IoT applications. The great load and variability of data processed there, the research-oriented personnel, and the funding these institutions can receive make IoT-health robotics assessment research possible (Yoon and Lee 2019). In the upcoming future, the cost of IoT-integrated devices is estimated to be trillions of dollars, besides the several limitations involving the quality of healthcare services, patient engagement, data security and privacy, health big data, and ethical aspects of the human factor (Evans 2011). Yet, security is still an open issue, and hence the growth in IoT-based context would add more challenging requirements.

Healthcare robotics is expected to redefine healthcare organizational culture. The organizational culture of a healthcare structure, from private practices to univer-sity hospitals, is equally important to the personnel and the equipment according to the Donabedian model of healthcare quality. Smart hospitals are the adequate infrastructure – or perhaps the adequate ecosystem – for robots. According to the Pan American Health Organization – WHO, smart healthcare facilities link their structural and operational safety with green interventions, at a reasonable cost-to-benefit ratio. Hence, when it comes to health robotics, smart healthcare facilities are expected to be renovated in terms of power supply, with a focus on green energy, structural improvements that will ensure the optimal storing of robots such as air-condition and humidity control systems, and network capacity and in terms of IoT and 5G infrastructure, among others. Such a reform will benefit patients and health-care personnel along with robots (Bedaf, Gelderblom, and De Witte 2015; Özdemir and Hekim 2018; Alaiad and Zhou 2014).

CONCLUSIONS

Health robotics enhances the quality of healthcare, improves healthcare workforce resilience, and brings significant contributions to research and education. With robots collecting information, IoT interconnection is vital to make this information available to healthcare providers. In the future, healthcare systems would adopt fur-ther developed and affordable technologies including IoT-integrated robotic systems that could operate easily in various settings and with various and challenging tasks. Hence, robots would take a key part in the fourth industrial revolutionary IoT tech-nology. Globally, several institutions and experts are working to address IoT imple-mentation and limitations, and enhancement of infrastructure, and standardization. The chapter discussed the perspective gains and obstacles of integrating robotics and the IoT in the health sector.

REFERENCES

Ackerman, Evan. 2018. "Cyberdyne's Medical Exoskeleton Strides to FDA Approval – IEEE Spectrum." *IEEE Spectrum: Technology, Engineering, and Science News.* January 23, 2018. https://spectrum.ieee.org/the-human-os/biomedical/devices/cyberdynes-medical- exoskeleton-strides-to-fda-approval.

Alaiad, Ahmad, and Lina Zhou. 2014. "The Determinants of Home Healthcare Robots Adoption: An Empirical Investigation." *International Journal of Medical Informatics* 83 (11): 825–840. doi: 10.1016/j.ijmedinf.2014.07.003.

Bakhru, Vik. 2017. "The Future of Medical Robotics: How Technology Will Improve Health Outcomes." December 7, 2017. https://www.beckershospitalreview.com/healthcare-information-technology/the-future-of-medical-robotics-how-technology-will-improve-health-outcomes.html.

Bandyopadhyay, Debasis, and Jaydip Sen. 2011. "Internet of Things: Applications and Challenges in Technology and Standardization." *Wireless Personal Communications* 58 (1): 49–69. doi: 10.1007/s11277-011-0288-5.

Bedaf, Sandra, Gert Jan Gelderblom, and Luc De Witte. 2015. "Overview and Categorization of Robots Supporting Independent Living of Elderly People: What Activities Do They Support and How Far Have They Developed." *Assistive Technology: The Official Journal of RESNA* 27 (2): 88–100. doi: 10.1080/10400435.2014.978916.

Bogue, Robert. 2009. "Exoskeletons and Robotic Prosthetics: A Review of Recent Developments." *Industrial Robot: An International Journal* 36 (5): 421–427. doi: 10.1108/01439910910980141.

Broadbent, Elizabeth, Ngaire Kerse, Kathryn Peri, Hayley Robinson, Chandimal Jayawardena, Tony Kuo, Chandan Datta, et al. 2016. "Benefits and Problems of Health-Care Robots in Aged Care Settings: A Comparison Trial." *Australasian Journal on Ageing* 35 (1): 23–29. doi: 10.1111/ajag.12190.

Butter, M., Arjan Rensma, J. van Boxsel, Sandy Kalisingh, Marian Schoone, Miriam Leis, Gert Jan Gelderblom, et al. 2008. "Robotics for Healthcare: Final Report." http://resolver.tudelft.nl/uuid:beddf38c-e88c-4d2a-8394-e7234d9b3e8a.

Cao, Hoang-Long, Pablo Gómez Esteban, Albert De Beir, Ramona Simut, Greet van de Perre, Dirk Lefeber, and Bram Vanderborght. 2017a. "A Survey on Behavior Control Architectures for Social Robots in Healthcare Interventions." *International Journal of Humanoid Robotics* 14 (4): 1750021. doi: 10.1142/S0219843617500219.

Cao, Hoang-Long, Pablo Gómez Esteban, Albert De Beir, Ramona Simut, Greet van de Perre, Dirk Lefeber, and Bram Vanderborght. 2017b. "A Collaborative Homeostatic-Based Behavior Controller for Social Robots in Human–Robot Interaction Experiments." *International Journal of Social Robotics* 9 (5): 675–690. doi: 10.1007/s12369-017-0405-z.

Chai, Peter R., Haipeng Zhang, Guruprasad D. Jambaulikar, Edward W. Boyer, Labina Shrestha, Loay Kitmitto, Paige G. Wickner, Hojjat Salmasian, and Adam B. Landman. 2019. "An Internet of Things Buttons to Measure and Respond to Restroom Cleanliness in a Hospital Setting: Descriptive Study." *Journal of Medical Internet Research* 21 (6). doi: 10.2196/13588.

Challacombe, Ben. 2013. "Ben Challacombe in Defence of Robots." *The Health Service Journal* 123 (6378): 16–17.

Dervaderics, János. 2007. "The Beginnings of Robotic Surgery – From the Roots Up to the Da Vinci Telemanipulator System." *Orvosi Hetilap* 148 (49): 2307–2313. doi: 10.1556/OH.2007.28225.

Evans, Dave. 2011. "How the Next Evolution of the Internet Is Changing Everything." Undefined. https://www.semanticscholar.org/paper/How-the-Next-Evolution-of-the- Internet-Is-Changing-Evans/e4342d4687233ae12aa689407f97502d87a9f27b.

Fracastoro, Gerolamo, Giuseppe Borzellino, Annalisa Castelli, and Paolo Fiorini. 2005. "Robotics in General Surgery: Personal Experience, Critical Analysis and Prospectives." *Chirurgia Italiana* 57 (6): 687–693.

Gopal, Gayatri, Clemens Suter-Crazzolara, Luca Toldo, and Werner Eberhardt. 2019. "Digital Transformation in Healthcare – Architectures of Present and Future Information Technologies." *Clinical Chemistry and Laboratory Medicine* 57 (3): 328–335. doi: 10.1515/cclm-2018-0658.

Gope, Prosanta, and Tzonelih Hwang. 2016. "BSN-Care: A Secure IoT-Based Modern Healthcare System Using Body Sensor Network." *IEEE Sensors Journal* 16 (5): 1. https://www.academia.edu/26272339/BSN-Care_A_Secure_IoT-based_Modern_Healthcare_System_Using_Body_Sensor_Network.

Grasso, Costantino. 2018. "Challenges and Advantages of Robotic Nursing Care: A Social and Ethical Analysis." *The Corporate Social Responsibility and Business Ethics Blog* (blog). June 26, 2018. https://corporatesocialresponsibilityblog.com/2018/06/26/robotic-nursing-care/.

Grifantini, Kristina. 2010. "Robotic Nurse Washes Human." *MIT Technology Review.* November 10, 2010. https://www.technologyreview.com/2010/11/10/199054/robotic-nurse-washes-human/.

Hax, Vinícius Alves, Nelson Lopes Duarte Filho, Silvia Silva da Costa Botelho, and Odorico Machado Mendizabal. 2013. "ROS as a Middleware to Internet of Things." *Journal of Applied Computing Research* 2 (2): 91–97. doi: 10.4013/jacr.2012.22.05.

Koh, Dong Hoon, Won Sik Jang, Jae Won Park, Won Sik Ham, Woong Kyu Han, Koon Ho Rha, and Young Deuk Choi. 2018. "Efficacy and Safety of Robotic Procedures Performed Using the Da Vinci Robotic Surgical System at a Single Institute in Korea: Experience with 10000 Cases." *Yonsei Medical Journal* 59 (8): 975–981. doi: 10.3349/ymj.2018.59.8.975.

Latif, Siddique, Junaid Qadir, Shahzad Farooq, and Muhammad Ali Imran. 2017. "How 5G Wireless (and Concomitant Technologies) Will Revolutionize Healthcare?" *Future Internet* 9 (4): 93. doi: 10.3390/fi9040093.

Lazarte, Maria. 2014. "Enter the First Cyborg-Type Robot." *ISO.* September 1, 2014. https://www.iso.org/cms/render/live/en/sites/isoorg/contents/news/2014/09/Ref1882.html.

Martinez, Dale. 2020. "Medical Robotic Systems Market 2020 – Global Leading Players." *Elmira Daily* (blog). June 18, 2020. https://elmiradaily.com/medical-robotic-systems-market-2020-global-leading-players-industry-updates-growth-factor-and-future-investments-by-forecast-to-2026/5483/.

Mittelstadt, Brent. 2017. "Ethics of the Health-Related Internet of Things: A Narrative Review." *Ethics and Information Technology* 19 (3): 157–175. doi: 10.1007/s10676-017-9426-4.

O'Brolcháin, Fiachra, Simone de Colle, and Bert Gordijn. 2019. "The Ethics of Smart Stadia: A Stakeholder Analysis of the Croke Park Project." *Science and Engineering Ethics* 25 (3): 737–769. doi: 10.1007/s11948-018-0033-5.

Özdemir, Vural, and Nezih Hekim. 2018. "Birth of Industry 5.0: Making Sense of Big Data with Artificial Intelligence, 'The Internet of Things' and Next-Generation Technology Policy." *OMICS: A Journal of Integrative Biology* 22 (1): 65–76. doi: 10.1089/omi.2017.0194.

Patel, Ankit R., Rajesh S. Patel, Navdeep M. Singh, and Faruk S. Kazi. 2017. "Vitality of Robotics in Healthcare Industry: An Internet of Things (IoT) Perspective." In *Internet of Things and Big Data Technologies for Next Generation Healthcare*, edited by Chintan Bhatt, Nilanjan Dey, and Amira S. Ashour, 91–109. Studies in Big Data. Cham: Springer International Publishing. doi: 10.1007/978-3-319-49736-5_5.

Psiha, Maria M., and Panayiotis Vlamos. 2017. "IoT Applications with 5G Connectivity in Medical Tourism Sector Management: Third-Party Service Scenarios." *Advances in Experimental Medicine and Biology* 989: 141–154. doi: 10.1007/978-3-319-57348-9_12.

Souppouris, Aaron. 2012. "Robotic Wheelchair Can Climb Steps, Traverse Uneven Surfaces, Turn on the Spot." *The Verge*. October 15, 2012. https://www.theverge.com/2012/10/15/3505406/robotic-wheelchair-stair-climbing-uneven-surfaces-concept-prototype.

Stefano, George B., and Richard M. Kream. 2018. "The Micro-Hospital: 5G Telemedicine-Based Care." *Medical Science Monitor Basic Research* 24 (July): 103–104. doi: 10.12659/MSMBR.911436.

Taylor, R.H. 2006. "A Perspective on Medical Robotics." *Proceedings of the IEEE* 94 (9): 1652–1664. doi: 10.1109/JPROC.2006.880669.

The Journal of mHealth. 2018. "How Robots are Changing Community Pharmacy." August 15, 2018. https://thejournalofmhealth.com/how-robots-are-changing-community- pharmacy/.

Tomlinson, Zachary. 2018. "15 Medical Robots that are Changing the World." October 11, 2018. https://interestingengineering.com/15-medical-robots-that-are-changing-the-world.

Toyota. 2019. "Toyota Launches Rehabilitation Assist Robot." November 28, 2019. https://tectales.com/bionics-robotics/toyota-has-announced-the-launch-of-its-new-welwalk-ww-2000-a-robot-designed-to-provide-rehabilitation-support-to-individuals-with-lower-limb-paralysis.html.

WHO. 2013. "World Health Report 2013: Research for Universal Health Coverage." *World Health Organization*. https://www.who.int/whr/en/.

Yoon, Seong No, and DonHee Lee. 2019. "Artificial Intelligence and Robots in Healthcare: What are the Success Factors for Technology-Based Service Encounters?" *International Journal of Healthcare Management* 12 (3): 218–225. doi: 10.1080/20479700.2018.1498220.

2 Microrobots and Nanorobots in the Refinement of Modern Healthcare Practices

Aditya Srivastava, Aparna Seth
and Kalpna Katiyar
Dr. Ambedkar Institute of Technology for Handicapped

CONTENTS

INTRODUCTION: WHAT ARE 'NANOROBOTS'?

In the December of 1959, Richard Feynman gave a lecture titled "There's Plenty of Room at the Bottom," in which he suggested the concept of nanoscale machinery constructed by the rearrangement of atoms in the desired manner and also the bold idea of surgical nano-machines, which can be "swallowed" to operate on the patient (Feynman 1960). This innovative idea caught the fancy of artists and scientists alike, and hence the field of nanotechnology was conceived. It has been found in various studies that nanoparticles have dramatically different properties as compared to their bulk forms and thus can be used for the best interests of humanity. In the field of medicine, dendrimers and quantum dots have been extensively used in disease diagnosis, enhancement in imaging, and even therapeutic purposes for diseases like cancer. However, we have minimal control over the traversal and functioning of these particles, which is a limitation to this technology.

To overcome the limitations and achieve what Feynman meant by "swallowing the surgeon," robots having nanoscale dimensions were designed. Based on the order of magnitude of their size, these robots are commonly known as "Microrobots" and "Nanorobots." These robots are not as structurally and functionally sophisticated as traditional robots, simply because of the extreme size constraint in their case. These machines are primarily molecular, atomic, or cellular (Manjunath and Kishore 2014), and the prime focus in their development is on their traversal as well as the manipulation or operation on the target. Furthermore, experts are striving to improve the communication algorithms among individuals (i.e., the swarming algorithms) as well as with an external controlling entity (Al-Hudhud 2012).

Even so, we still need to overcome specific challenges for the successful development of nanorobots in medicine. These challenges may range from issues related to power, mobility, and communication to specific problems related to biocompatibility and immunogenicity (Elbaz and Willner 2012; Kostarelos 2010). All of these aspects, along with the prospective applications of nanorobots, have been discussed in detail herein.

TYPES OF NANOROBOTS

Nanotechnology is a multidisciplinary field of science that accesses considerable involvement of areas related to computer science, physics, chemistry, and biology for the prototype development of new devices and machines. Depending on the landscapes mentioned earlier and the nature of nanorobots, there are two types of nano-machines studied so far, which are:

- **Bio-nanorobots**: Biological entities such as biomolecules, DNA, RNA, protein, flagellar motor, and mitochondria are performing their specified functions since the emergence of life, consequently controlling excellent outcomes (Whitesides 2001). Bio-nanobots can be synthesized either by manipulating the size of such biomolecules or by self-assembly. Bio-nanobots exhibit various properties like self-replication, healing, adaptability, life, and intelligence. These are either naturally occurring molecular machines or ultimately created from natural components such as molecular motors, cilia, or cell components (Satir 1999; Oiwa 2003; Tyreman and Molloy 2003). They can produce driving forces through chemical or catalytic reactions happening within the cellular component for propulsion and motion. Obtaining a bio-nanorobot with natural sensors, transmission elements, motor, propeller, and controller would be a highly efficient and reliable approach. Nanorobotic devices are further categorized into protein-based molecular machines and DNA-based molecular tools (Ummat et al. 2016).
  1. **Protein-based molecular machines**: Proteins are versatile biomolecules, which show compatible interactions with other biomolecules. They also possess the self-assembling property and are responsible for performing numerous physiological functions (AZoNano 2017). The positioning of individual protein and protein complexes are the two most important aspects to be considered while utilizing proteins as nano-machines. The ATP synthase complex is one of the most common

examples of a protein-based molecular machine at the nanoscale, also known as 'a true nano-sized rotatory motor,' applicable in controlling mechanical motions and powering the rotation of a nano-sized propeller (Soong et al. 2000). Other such examples include kinesin, myosin, dynein, and flagella molecular motors functioning at the nanoscale (Ummat et al. 2016). In addition to this, proteins in response to external stimuli such as pH undergo different conformational changes, which in turn would yield variation in designs of nano-machines (Strong 2004).

2. **DNA-based molecular machines**: Fabrication of DNA nano-machines of different designs as well as altered shape, size, and spatial addressability to dynamically interact with each other for generating logical outputs and establishing biomedical applications is known as DNA Origami (Amir et al. 2014). DNA nanobots are constructed using natural, versatile scaffolds of mechanical molecular devices. This confers on them various properties like the ability to respond to external triggers and recomposing their assembly for payload delivery (Douglas, Bachelet, and Church 2012). It serves as a targeted drug delivery system, pH-mapping probe, and imaging probe designed for sensing, actuating, and enhanced functioning at the nanoscale (S. Li et al. 2018). A DNA-based nanorobot composed of DNA fragments has been designed at the ITMO University to detect, locate, and destroy cancer cells by blocking the production of disease-related proteins and cleaving bonds of the pathogenic RNA strand. In addition, by injecting these bots in mice, scientists are trying to perform vascular occlusion, which can help treat human breast cancer tumors. In this method, blood clotting is initiated in *de-novo* vessels of the tumor, thus cutting off the blood supply and leading to the death of cancer cells (Devasena Umai, Brindha Devi, and Thiruchelvi 2018; S. Li et al. 2018).

3. **Chemical-based molecular machines**: Certain mechanically interlocked molecular arrangements like pseudorotaxanes, rotaxanes, and catenanes have been proposed to be used as molecular motors, switches, and shuttles (Balzani, Gómez-López, and Stoddart 1998). Cyclodextrin, a cyclic oligosaccharide, is a crucial constituent of these supra-molecular frameworks employed in the development of micro or nano-level machines (Harada 2001). All these organic compounds are capable of charging themselves with the light, electron, and chemical energy to guide their motion within the cell. This conversion of chemical energy into mechanical energy (or change in the ionization state of the cell because of the transfer of hydrogen atoms between two organisms) is the cause of rotatory motion and movement of chemical-based nanodevices (Amendola et al. 2001). Other than this, nucleotide hydrolysis, ligand binding, Brownian changes of polymerizing filaments, and fluctuating cellular environment are some types of energy-producing standards that provide energy to biological springs and ratchets for initiating spring-like action in *Vorticella*, a unicellular organism, also permitting its motility (Mahadevan and Matsudaira 2000).

- **Artificial nanorobots**: These nanorobots are composed of a non-toxic, biocompatible elemental material that degrades itself within the body after accomplishing the set goal (Li et al. 2019; Loukanov et al. 2016). Perhaps, such specific, reprogrammable, and autonomously fabricated nanoelectromechanical devices mimic the biological systems or mechanisms to work as per the physiological processes and store, deliver, and release payload to the targeted site due to external triggers (Büther et al. 2017; Dressler and Kargl 2012). To power artificial nanorobots, their design depends upon two fundamental principles, i.e., photo- or magnetic activation, to manufacture light-activated nano-sized impeller and magnetic nano vehicles (Loukanov, Gagov, and Nakabayashi 2020). Other elementary components of artificial/ engineered nanorobots include onboard sensors, propeller, controller, capacitor/detector/actuator, camera, magnet, fluorescence system, camera, molecular computer, and manipulator indispensable to aping the biological nano-machines (Requicha 2003; Mitthra et al. 2016; Cavalcanti et al. 2008). Currently, researchers are working on the development of nanobots to take advantage of the area of hematology to transport oxygen inside the body after severing contusion artificially. Respirocytes and clottocytes are two hypothetical nanorobots engineered to imitate red blood cells and natural platelets, respectively, applied to alleviate the patient immediately. Due to the advancement in the field, ardent exploration, and rapid development, nanobots will soon find their application in the fields of health care, environmental remediation, detoxification, biohazard defense, and many more shortly.

FABRICATION TECHNIQUES AND MATERIALS

As stated earlier, micro- and nanorobots show tremendous potential in biomedical applications. However, to function desirably, specific challenges need to be addressed. The prime hurdle among them is the issue of mobility, which is due to the dramatically different medium properties that these nano-machines experience. At sizes as small as the micro and nanoscale, the features of the fluid medium in which these particles are designed to swim are significantly altered because of the predominance of intermolecular as well as liquid drag forces and the negligibility of the inertial forces (Qiu and Nelson 2015). This change in properties manifests as a subsequent decrease in the Reynolds number of the medium, i.e., the medium appears to be highly viscous (Abbott et al. 2009). The reason behind this is the increase in the surface area-to-volume ratio (Sengupta, Ibele, and Sen 2012). Also, any minuscule particles or entities placed in such media are bound to show negligible displacement due to reciprocal motion. Since the movement necessarily needs to be non-reciprocal for the robots to traverse the complex media in a biological system, they have to be individually tailored and designed for this purpose (Nelson and Peyer 2014). Furthermore, the traversal in a medium with such properties is an energy-expensive affair, which means that the nano-machines must be capable of harnessing as well as harvesting energy from the surrounding physical or chemical energy sources (Sengupta, Ibele, and Sen 2012; Guix, Mayorga-Martinez, and Merkoçi 2014; Dey and Sen 2017; Wang and Pumera 2018; Li, Rozen, and Wang 2016; Katuri et al. 2017).

In the case of nanorobots that are to be used for applications in clinical and biomedical purposes, it must be ensured that the material used for the fabrication must be completely biocompatible and non-toxic. If not so, then the material must at least be biodegradable so that it can be easily removed from the body after its purpose is served (Lin et al. 2016). Various independent groups have been exploring different materials for the fabrication of nanorobots for specialized applications (Gao and Wang 2014; Li et al. 2017; Wang and Pumera 2015; Chen et al. 2018). An example of such materials is mesoporous silica, which is entirely biodegradable under certain conditions (Ma et al. 2015, 2016), and its non-toxicity in human cell lines has been established. Some groups have also reported nanomotor apparatus made of a material that disintegrates in the course of traversal of the nanobots, such that they completely dissolve into removable forms once their cargo is delivered. Such nanorobots simultaneously address the issues related to fueled propulsion as well as biocompatibility (Gao, Pei, and Wang 2012; Mou et al. 2013).

Various fabrication techniques are used in the manufacturing of nanorobots, depending on the material constitution. In the case of biohybrid nanorobots, these techniques may differ significantly. The primary methods are described as follows:

- **Self-scrolling method**: In this method, the material, which may be a magnetic metal (Bell et al. 2007) or a biological substance (Schuerle et al. 2012), is curled up using thin-film deposition or mono-crystalline thin-film deposition methods, while simultaneously manipulating the curvature and the three-dimensional (3D) orientation of the material. This method is mainly used for the production of helical nanorobots and microswimmers (X. Z. Chen et al. 2017).
- **Glancing angle deposition (GLAD)**: In this method, the substrate is continuously rotated, such that the magnetic material gets deposited according to the deposition/glancing angle, hence resulting in the formation of a curved nanostructure (Qiu and Nelson 2015). Many helical nano-machines have been fabricated using this procedure (X. Z. Chen et al. 2017).
- **Template-assisted electrodeposition method and biotemplated synthesis**: In this method, a template material (which may be of biological origin, e.g., plant vascular tissue) is used to fabricate microswimmers by the electrodeposition of a manufacturing material. The structural properties of the nanobots thus produced depend mainly on the characteristics of the template and can be controlled accordingly (Gao et al. 2014). Nanobots like flexible swimmers and micro diggers are also synthesized using these methods (X. Z. Chen et al. 2017).
- **Direct laser writing method**: This is a 3D laser-based lithographic method, which comes with the added benefit of the freedom to create arbitrary shaped 3D structures. In this method, a laser beam is used on a photoresist mounted on a suitable base to develop it desirably. The designed nanostructures are then coated with magnetic materials through electron-beam evaporative deposition (Qiu and Nelson 2015).

- **Hydrothermal carbonization**: This method is employed for the mass-production of randomly shaped nanostructures. It is a quick and inexpensive procedure and can be efficiently conducted (Vach et al. 2015).
- **Molecular self-assembly**: In some instances, biomolecules like nucleic acids are programmed using sequence-specific interactions (Bogue 2010) for self-assembly to ensure utmost biocompatibility. This is often referred to as "DNA Origami" (Tørring et al. 2011) and has been used for the production of "DNA walkers" and clam-shaped DNA nanobots, which are also known as "nubots" (Bogue 2010). DNA nanobots have been instrumental in site-specific targeting and drug delivery after suitable functionalization (Elbaz and Willner 2012).

In some instances, naturally occurring biological entities have also been harnessed and customized for usage as nanorobotic machinery. This approach also ensures versatility along with complete biocompatibility, as has been displayed in the case of the Chaperonin GroEL machinery (Sim and Aida 2017).

SIZE, STRUCTURE, AND DESIGN

In these trending times of miniaturization, nano-machines have come up with staggering features reassuring all attributes, essentially precision, sustainability, affectivity, and speed (Agrahari et al. 2020). The ultrafine particles, ranging from 1 to 100 nm, are obliging in presenting a large surface area-to-volume ratio, which successively illustrates more enhanced behavior compared to their bulk size. Nanorobots are mechanical or electromechanical submicroscopic devices fundamentally constructed of atomic-sized particles using methods like self-assembly (Saxena et al. 2015). Manipulation of particles at each level of the assembly plays a crucial role in their positioning and orientation. The structure of a nanorobot is categorical, as per its function to be performed, aimed at theranostics, imaging, and drug delivery (Mertz 2018). The exterior of the device needs to be smooth enough to prevent any kind of interference in body functions as well as the immune system (Saxena et al. 2015). In addition to it, the carbon surface provides strength while the motor attached to it generates a remarkable torque and decides the direction of movement (Senanayake, Sirisinghe, and Mun 2007). Designing is majorly based on the signal processing technology, navigation, recognition, and controller to handle networks (Liu and Nakano 2012). Biohybrid, chemically powered, and physically powered nanorobots are the three types of powered nanorobots that can harvest energy through different methods to potentially drive into the body. Therefore, these nanorobots work at an atomic, molecular, and cellular level (Soto and Chrostowski 2018; Mallouk and Sen 2009).

Because of this science being rather recent and advanced, and due to a lack of expertise, simulation and modeling are imperative for its devising. Assembly automation and instrumentation are done via a practical approach with an advanced computer-aided manufacturing methodology that embraces software platforms like 3Dstudio MAX software, Nanorobot Control Design (NCD) software, and so on to simulate and design nanobots (Senanayake, Sirisinghe, and Mun 2007; Cavalcanti, Hogg, and Shirinzadeh 2006).

Several prototypes designed primarily based on hallmark characteristics point-edly power, motion control, proficiency, multivariance, and functionality of nanoro-bots include nanoswimmers, nano-sized transducers, 3D DNA nano-machines, sperm-like nanobots, and surface walkers (Li et al. 2019; Wilson 2018). Some of these have been described as follows:

- **Nanoswimmers**: These nanorobots are composites of a ferromagnetic material such as gold, silver, and platinum to ensure the biocompatible nature and facilitate the functionalization of various biological substances (Laocharoensuk, Burdick, and Wang 2008; Manesh, Balasubramanian, and Wang 2010). It requires either a magnetic field or different chemicals for generating thrust force and controlling movement to simulate the actuation of flagellated bacteria (Kotesa, Rathore, and Sharma 2013; Mallouk and Sen 2009). Certain imaging technologies employed for tracking, imaging, and localizing the nanoswimmers in such dynamic environment of the body involve optical monitoring, magnetic imaging, ultrasound imaging, X-ray imaging, and fluorescence imaging (Zhang et al. 2009; Dahmen, Wortmann, and Fatikow 2012; Mavroidis and Ferreira 2013; Ullrich et al. 2013; Pané et al. 2019). Nanoswimmers can be of the following general types:
  1. **Helical Swimmers**: These micro- and nanorobots are fabricated in a heli-cal fashion, such that they can be easily actuated with the help of a rotating magnetic field. They have been studied in great detail (Qiu and Nelson 2015; Nelson and Peyer 2014) and show great promise in the targeted delivery of drugs and other compounds. Helical nanobots have even been reported to transport sperm cells to the external layers of the ovum *in vitro*.
  2. **Flexible swimmers**: This is an umbrella term for all those nanorobots, which have been designed to have flexible bodies, tails, or even wholly bendable bodies (X. Z. Chen et al. 2017). Periodic magnetic fields also propel these and primarily depend on the undulations of their flexible bodies during traversal. These nanorobots have been designed to mimic the swimming patterns of various eukaryotic cells. Some biohybrid specimens of this kind even rely on actual microbes attached to their bodies for propulsion (Carlsen et al. 2014).
- **Nano-transducer**: Also known as an actuating nano-transducer, the tini-est engine invented so far could quickly move inside the cellular body for diagnosis and treatment. It possesses the ability to predict the atmosphere. It can provide a variety of information when optimized accordingly—mainly composed of gold and some temperature-reactive polymers, which when heated by a laser collect an ample amount of electric energy within seconds. These are simple, fast, biocompatible, energy-efficient, and optically pow-ered nanorobots (Malewar 2016).
- **3D DNA nano-machines**: These are self-assembled and self-powered nano-machines with high movement efficacy (Wen et al. 2019). A DNA nano-machine is modeled along the lines of biological systems or bio-molecular machines, and it can alter its framework due to external trig-gers when necessary (Bath and Turberfield 2007). The 3D triangular

prism nano-machines can quickly drive into living cells for performing pH sensing, sensitive detection, and imaging by generating fluorescence (Zhou et al. 2019).

- **Sperm-like nanobots**: These can be either artificial cells, powered by chemicals, ultrasonics, and magnetic field, or natural cells, possessing self-propelling motors with some alterations, to function like a robot. Moreover, research scientists are attempting to formulate a hybrid by blending both artificial and natural aspects to procure a nanorobot with high efficiency and effectiveness (Kwon 2018). The purpose of their fabrication is to load drugs and travel through the female reproductive tract for treating both male and female infertility problems, uterus cancer, cervical cancer, and other gynecological diseases (Servick 2016; Nelson 2008).

- **Surface walkers**: In truth, all nanobots (which may belong to any structural category or design) that traverse close to any biological surface can be called surface walkers. The primary mode of traversal is by rolling or tumbling, with or without any actual contact with the surface. These may be of any shape or size (for example, Janus spheres or nano-beads) and are instrumental in carrying the cargo with the help of a vortex produced because of their motion (Zhang et al. 2010).

In addition to these, there are some other examples like the plant-based 'microdaggers,' which can be employed to perform surgical operations on individual cells (Srivastava et al. 2016). Microbots having magnetic cilia-like structures all over their bodies (Kim et al. 2016), or even randomly shaped structures with speeds comparable to helical swimmers (Vach et al. 2015), can also be used for this purpose.

MOBILITY, COMMUNICATION, AND SWARMING

The presently developed nanorobots show tremendous promise in the targeted operation and delivery of a cargo. However, there are certain functional aspects, which are crucial for the efficient and desirable functioning of nanorobots. They are described in the following.

PROPULSION AND MOBILITY

As stated earlier, nanobots used for biomedical applications should be able to traverse through a wide variety of fluid media, which may be merely homogeneous or even heterogeneous mixed media (Nelson and Peyer 2014). Furthermore, the nanoscale dimensions of the machinery make it all the more difficult to travel through such media, as the viscous drag and other molecular forces are predominant instead of the traditional macro-scale inertial forces (Bogue 2010; Qiu and Nelson 2015). These difficulties cannot be resolved by fabrication and designing solutions alone. Therefore, the said nanobots must be capable of utilizing energy from the various sources available in their surroundings (Sengupta, Ibele, and Sen 2012). Thus, powering the propulsion mechanism of these nano-machines becomes a rather challenging task, which is worsened by the fact that wiring and circuit designing are not possible at such scales. Furthermore, the propulsion also has to be directional and target-oriented to increase efficiency and specificity. These properties can be achieved using external stimuli (such as electrical or magnetic fields or ultrasound waves) or internal factors (like pH, temperature, and chemical nature of the traversing medium) (Ma and Sánchez 2017).

Among all the energy transmission strategies being analyzed nowadays, magnetic transmission has emerged as the most promising mode of energy transmission, as it does not depend on conducting media. It is also harmless when used on biological subjects. Furthermore, low-intensity magnetic fields have proved to be pivotal in guiding stray nanorobots, which may or may not be self-propelled along the directed course. Many groups, including the one at the University of Waterloo, have been involved in the study of magnetic propulsion for use in microbots for minute surgical operations as well as highly targeted cargo delivery (Bogue 2010). There are undoubtedly other strategies, like the use of ultrasound waves to guide the motion of nanorobots for the successful delivery of GFP siRNA (Ma and Sánchez 2017). Also, some groups have worked on light-powered nano-machines. However, their use in biological systems is still a subject of debate, as the use of high-power UV or infrared radiations for the propulsion can prove to be harmful to the living systems (Xuan et al. 2016; Dai et al. 2016; C. Chen et al. 2017).

Various propulsion and actuation strategies that are being examined for use in nanorobots have been described as follows:

- **Catalyst-based bubble propulsion**: Certain nano-machines have been designed generally as tubular nanostructures (Gao et al. 2011), which have a catalytic substance incorporated in their centers (Katuri et al. 2017). This catalyst can convert specific chemical substrates like hydrogen peroxide (Sengupta, Ibele, and Sen 2012) into their constituents, releasing bubbles, which result in propulsion due to the recoil of the bubbles. Furthermore, factors like surfactants (Wang, Zhao, and Pumera 2014) and curve radius (Magdanz et al. 2014) are also known to influence the stability of the bubbles produced. However, the fuels used by these nanomotors are often toxic to the biological system and may cause oxidative stress (Katuri et al. 2017; Ma and Sánchez 2017), which is why their use for biomedical purposes is still under consideration.
- **Enzyme-based propulsion**: This mode of propulsion is more biocompatible because there is no dependence on toxic fuels. In this case, the surface of the nanobots is differentially infused with enzymes like catalase, urease, or glucose oxidase (Ma et al. 2015, 2016; Dey et al. 2015; Abdelmohsen et al. 2016; Bunea et al. 2015), which enables them to use biologically/physiologically available fuels like glucose and urea for their propulsion (Ma and Sánchez 2017). These nanobots are generally fabricated as Janus spheres, nanorods, and nanotubes, and their functionality has been demonstrated *in vivo* (Katuri et al. 2017).
- **Self-electrophoretic propulsion**: These nanorobots are created using bimetallic designing schemes, i.e., using two metals, generally as nanorods or other dynamically feasible shapes. In the presence of an ionic medium or a medium that can undergo catalytic ionization by the particular metals,

the nanorods develop an electric field across themselves due to the electro-chemical interactions of the medium. This new electric field results in the production of a "slip velocity," which is responsible for the propulsion of the device (Paxton et al. 2004; Fournier-Bidoz et al. 2005). Significant improve-ments have been made in this propulsion technique (Liu and Sen 2011). Still, the versatility of this type of nanomotors is questionable because of their dependence on the ionic characteristics of the medium, which are not very uniform in this case.

- **Diffusion-based propulsion**: This is an enhanced version of self-electrophoretic propulsion. In this case, a difference in the diffusivity of cations and anions causes the formation of a net electric field, which propels the nanorobots forward. The propelling force is also enhanced by the devel-opment of osmotic pressure because of the concentration gradient of ions (Sengupta, Ibele, and Sen 2012). Since this also affects the nano-environment of the nanobots, which in a way acts as a chemical signal system, it results in a push or pull exerted on the nearby particles, which can be considered as a primitive form of swarm-behavior (M. Ibele, Mallouk, and Sen 2009; M. E. Ibele et al. 2010).

  Diffusion-based propulsion may also occur due to osmotic pressures developed from the concentration gradients of non-electrolytes, depend-ing upon whether the particle–solute interaction is attractive or repulsive. Specially functionalized Janus spheres called "microspiders" have been designed *in vivo*, which propel themselves through non-electrolytic diffu-sion (Pavlick et al. 2011).

- **Self-propelling biohybrids**: These are the most biologically compatible and promising nanobots, designed for reliable propulsion using pre-existent natural systems. In some instances, nanobots are clubbed with flagellated bacteria to achieve thrust through flagellar motion (Carlsen et al. 2014). In some cases, the bacteria used are magnetotactic. Hence, they enable the magnetic actuation of the nanorobots (Martel 2011), along with magnetic resonance imaging for real-time monitoring of the traversal of the nanobots. The magnetotactic actuation of bacterial nanobots, along with the variation in the behavior of the flagellar machinery in response to environmental stimuli (addition of chemicals like DMSO and ethylene glycol in the media), has been studied in detail (Ali et al. 2017). In addition to bacteria, various "spermbots" have been developed using bull or other mammalian spermatozoa, which show great potential in the targeting of nanobots, with or without external guidance, and even in the treatment for infertility (Khalil et al. 2014; Magdanz et al. 2015, 2016; Medina-Sánchez et al. 2016).

All these propulsion mechanisms, along with some external accessory guiding forces like electric, magnetic, thermal, or photonic fields, can be used for the effective con-trol of the trajectory of the nanorobots. However, all the demonstrations to date are merely proof-of-concept and need to be improved further before being implemented into actual biomedical applications (Ma and Sánchez 2017).

COMMUNICATION AND THE SWARMING BEHAVIOR

A factor that is crucial for the improvement of performance and biomedical applicability of nanorobots is the development of communication among neighboring entities, as well as with an external controlling body. A sound communication system ensures that the nanomotors can be guided and controlled along their course of action and can work as a collective unit instead of numerous scattered entities. This cooperative approach, which is known as "swarming," has been explored significantly in the course of the I-SWARM (Intelligent Small-World Autonomous Robots for Micromanipulation) research project funded by the EU (Bogue 2010). A coordinated operation by nanorobots for any biomedical application can prove to be far more superior to any catheter-based techniques that are in use today. However, swarming and synchronization have only been achieved *in vivo*, and practical implementation is yet to be achieved.

To gain synchronization among individual nanobots, communication using low-frequency acoustic signals has been explored by Hogg and Freitas Jr., who also conducted an in-depth mathematical study of the acoustic characteristics of both nanobots and tissues (Hogg and Freitas Jr. 2012). Furthermore, the removal of cholesterol plaques using nanorobots coordinated by both centralized and decentralized approaches has been successfully explored by Al-Hudhud, who also proposed detailed algorithms for both approaches (Al-Hudhud 2012).

APPLICATION OF NANOROBOTS IN MEDICINE

Scientific minds are nowadays more inclined toward achieving a more straightforward, cost-effective, efficient, simple, fast, and more accurate technology to encompass all pitfalls faced while handling complicated and expensive devices. Robotic systems principally focus on sensing, interacting, manipulating, and transforming stuff, which in turn affects the world on the whole. The formulation of nanorobots has the potential to impressively change a large number of fields such as agriculture, energy, environment, electronics, and especially biomedicine and health care (Torney et al. 2007; Zhang, Yu, and Braun 2011; Jarosz et al. 2011).

By employing nanodevices in health care, experts are working toward achieving a better means of early detection, testing, and treatment of diseases to prevent toxicity in the body. Because of their propensity to drive through biological non-Newtonian fluids, this technology is employed for targeted drug delivery, simplification of complex surgical procedures, stress-free biosensing and detoxification, processes that usually rely on systemic circulation for the treatment of infected cells or tissues, diseases, and defects (Katuri et al. 2017).

Some applications of nanorobots in biomedical sciences are as follows:

1. **Surgical nanorobots**: When introduced through the vascular system or cavities, these could navigate throughout as well as get to every hard-to-reach location within the body subsequently, act as an on-site surgeon, and reduce the difficulties faced during severe complex surgical cases (Lanfranco et al. 2004; Barbash and Glied 2010). All this is made possible only by introducing microgrippers. An external controlling entity (a human surgeon or a computer)

can externally program them with high precision, flexibility, and control. Besides this, such surgical nanobots (Figure 2.1a and 2.1b) can convey timed signals to other cells to sleep, die, or regenerate through the logic gates of AND, OR, and XOR built within the system (Spendlove 2014).

2. **Sensors**: Easy surface functionalization of an analyte with bioreceptors enables nanorobots to sense and diagnose anomalies, which further isolates biological targets and increases the binding efficiency, sensitivity, and speed of biological assays (Figure 2.2a–c) (Wang 2016). Therefore, they can also be used for diagnosis as detection, isolation, therapeutic, and imaging agents. Some nanorobot sensors have been developed using various analytes like pore proteins of *Staphylococcus aureus* alpha-hemolysin, cholera toxin, and photoreceptive polypeptides like azobenzene or spiropyran (Mazumder, Biswas, and Majee 2020). Scientists have used such nanorobots to monitor neural connection patterns through minimally invasive approaches (Martins, Erlhagen, and Freitas 2012) and for the triangulation of cancerous cell masses (Dolev, Narayanan, and Rosenblit 2019).

3. **Nanorobotic dentifrices**: Developments in nanotechnology are relevant in maintaining oral hygiene, cavity preparation and restoration, repair and reposting teeth, inducing anesthesia, esthetic dentistry, and dentin hypersensitivity. Solutions containing nanorobots can be used as a mouthwash. Such solutions are capable of removing dental plaques, tartar, bacteria, and other organic matter by converting them into harmless vapors (Mazumder, Biswas, and Majee 2020; Padovani et al. 2015). They are exceptionally efficient because of their ability to reach minute crevices that are usually inaccessible as shown in Figure 2.3.

4. **Biomimetic nanobots**: These are nanoscale robotic systems that mimic biochemical processes or signatures and, in turn, sustain their biocompatibility when introduced into a biological system. Researchers are attempting to develop biohybrid nanorobots composed of a gold nanowire coated with both red blood cells and platelet membranes to achieve two different results

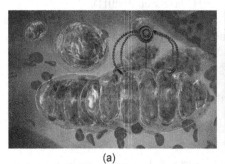 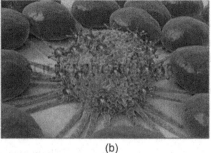

(a)   (b)

FIGURE 2.1 Surgical nanorobots: (a) nanodocs in precision surgery (swallow the surgeon), mobile microgrippers. (Four Ways We Can "Swallow the Doctor") (Nanodocs, the medical nanorobots by Brady Hartman.) (b) Nanorobots targeting a tumor site. (Nanorobots a Future Device for Diagnosis and Treatment by Sarath Kumar S., Beena P. Nasim, and Elessy Abraham.)

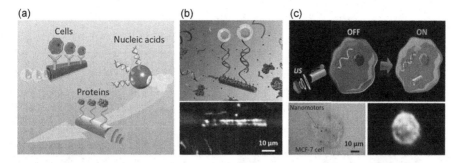

FIGURE 2.2 Micro/nanorobots for sensing. (a) Functionalization of a micro/nanorobot with different bioreceptors toward biosensing of target analytes, including cells, proteins, and nucleic acids. (b) ssDNA-functionalized microrockets for selective hybridization and isolation of nucleic acids. (c) Specific intracellular detection of miRNA in intact cancer cells using ultrasound (US) propulsion. (Li, Jinxing, et al. "Micro/Nanorobots for Biomedicine: Delivery, Surgery, Sensing, and Detoxification." *Science Robotics* 2.4 (2017).)

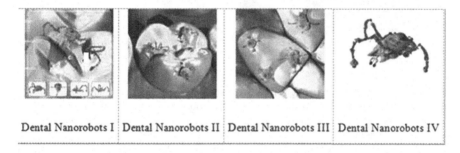

FIGURE 2.3 Medical nanobots capable of repairing the various tissues of the teeth and gums will bring new dimensions to dental care. (Gopal Reddy, N. "Nanotechnology Use in Medicine." *Journal of Evolution of Medical and Dental Sciences* 3.68, December 08 (2014): 14683–14693. doi: 10.14260/jemds/2014/3971.)

at the same time. In this direction, de Ávila et al. have developed specific hybrid biomembrane-functionalized nanobots that are capable of triangulating and disposing of pathogens and other immunogenic threats (de Ávila et al. 2018). Furthermore, teams at the University of California, San Diego, have developed ultrasound-powered robots that can perform detoxification of the whole body along their way (J. Li et al. 2018) (Figure 2.4).

5. **Therapeutic agents**: The probabilities of treating cancer, genetic diseases, diabetes, atherosclerosis, gout cerebral aneurysm, and oral disease have tremendously increased over time in the era of nanotechnology (Ahmad et al. 2014; Patil et al. 2016). In this case, nanorobots are a promising agent to carry a payload for targeted drug delivery with equal distribution of drugs at a specific site. Nano-sized robots have been employed for direct intravascular therapy, nanogene therapy, and tumor therapy, yielding much more sounding results (Sivasankar and Durairaj 2012). Nanobots show great

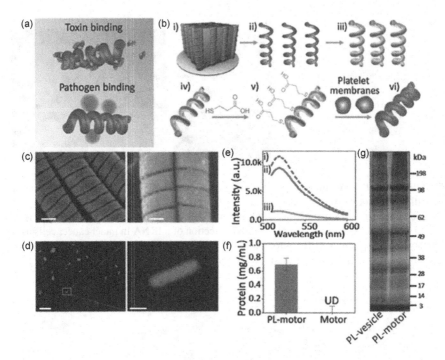

FIGURE 2.4 Biomimetic nanobots. (a) Schematic of PL-motors for binding and isolation of platelet-specific toxins and pathogens. (b) Preparation of PL-motors: (i) Pd/Cu co-electro-deposition in a polycarbonate membrane with a pore size of 400 nm. (ii) Dissolution of Cu using nitric acid and release of the helical Pd nanostructures. (iii) Deposition of Ni/Au bilayer on the Pd helical nanostructure. (iv) Collection of the helical nanostructures. (v) Modification of the bare helical nanomotor surface with 3-mercaptopropionic acid (MPA). (vi) Fusion of platelet-membrane-derived vesicles (denoted "PL vesicles") to the MPA-modified surface of the helical nanomotor. (c) Representative SEM images of the fabricated bare nanomotors without platelet coating (left) and PL motors (right). Scale bars, 100 nm. (d) Fluorescent images of PL motors covered with rhodamine-labeled platelet membranes. Scale bars, 20 μm (left) and 1 μm (right). (e) Fluorescence quenching assay to determine the platelet membrane coverage of the PL motors. Fluorescence spectra of (i) FITC-thiol only, (ii) FITC-thiol and PL motor mixture, and (iii) FITC-thiol and bare motor mixture. (f) The measured weight of protein content on bare motors and PL motors (both 10 mg/mL) stored in 1X PBS at 4°C for 24 hours. Error bars represent the standard deviation from three different measurements. UD, undetectable. (g) Sodium dodecyl sulfate polyacrylamide gel electrophoresis (SDS-PAGE) analysis of proteins present on the PL vesicles and the PL motors. The samples were run at equal protein content and stained with Coomassie Blue. (Li, Jinxing, et al. "Biomimetic Platelet-Camouflaged Nanorobots for Binding and Isolation of Biological Threats." *Advanced Materials* 30.2 (2018): 1704800.)

potential in the diagnosis and treatment of cancer (Venkatesan and Jolad 2010). Particular acoustic nanobots have also shown potential therapeutic usage in disease with the help of low-frequency acoustic pulses and even positron emission tomography (Hogg and Freitas Jr. 2012; Maheswari et al. 2018). Biohybrid nanorobots have also immensely contributed to the province of therapeutics (Akin et al. 2007) and are shown in Figure 2.5.

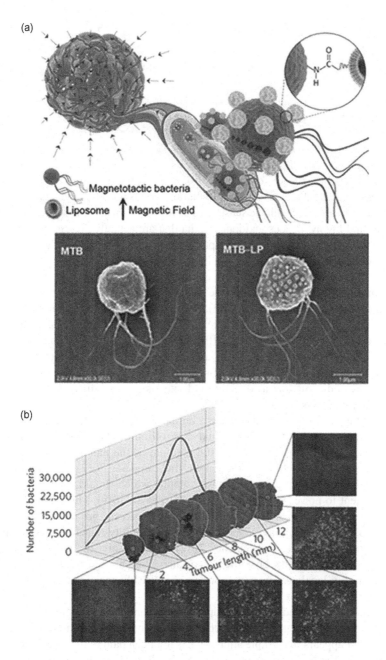

FIGURE 2.5 Nanorobots as therapeutic agents for delivery usage. (a) Schematic illustration and SEM of a biohybrid nanorobot including a magnetotactic bacteria loaded with liposomes. (b) Fluorescent images of transverse tumor sections illustrating the biohybrid robot distribution and population inside the tumor. (Soto, Fernando, and Robert Chrostowski. "Frontiers of Medical Micro/Nanorobotics: In Vivo Applications and Commercialization Perspectives Toward Clinical Uses." *Frontiers in Bioengineering and Biotechnology* 6 (2018): 170.)

CHALLENGES, CONSTRAINTS, AND LOOSE ENDS

As far as the technological advances are concerned, nanobots do offer a most radical approach that has the potential to revolutionize healthcare. However, the technique is still in its initial stages of infancy, and the realization of this technology still needs research and innovative diligence to achieve desirable functionality (Li et al. 2019). Furthermore, there are many challenges yet to overcome, for example, the fabrication-related and powering-related constraints, which still baffle many experts. Most materials (Bumb, Bhaskar, and Punia 2013) and fuels like hydrogen peroxide (Katuri et al. 2017; Ma and Sánchez 2017) that are used for the fabrication of the nanobots may initiate biocompatibility issues (Kostarelos 2010), which can lead to further complications when applied in actual scenarios. A novel solution for this issue is enzymatic propulsion, which uses biologically available substances as fuels, but this is only successful experimentally, and highly viscous and ionic media that are actually present in a biological system are impossible to traverse in the present situations (Ma and Sánchez 2017).

As individual *in-vivo* examinations have shown, a blindfolded approach without any form of coordination, or at least communication, between the nanobots in a swarm may have crippling effects on the overall efficacy of the operation (Al-Hudhud 2012; Bumb, Bhaskar, and Punia 2013). A catalog of supremely complicated desirable properties (Manjunath and Kishore 2014), which are hard to achieve because of the size constraint, leads to further difficulties in fabrication. This and the fact that the uniform fabrication of structurally and dimensionally same nanoparticles is not possible, or practically feasible on a large scale, are the reasons for the difference in efficiency and actuation, as different individuals respond differently to the same stimuli (Bumb, Bhaskar, and Punia 2013).

Medical nanodevices must be able to communicate and exchange signals among each other, as well as with an external controlling entity (Hogg and Freitas Jr. 2012). Also, the molecular forces of the medium at the nanoscale are supremely dominant over the inertial forces (Sengupta, Ibele, and Sen 2012). Considering these facts, nanobots require a constant power supply, which should be quick and suitably sufficient to power the entire operation (Li et al. 2019). This is easy as far as proof-of-concept demonstrations in the lab are concerned, but the current options may fail to suffice. They may even trigger biocompatibility-related issues in the case of non-natural fuels (Ma and Sánchez 2017). Furthermore, the proposed acoustic signaling mechanisms also pose the risk of disrupting normal tissue physiology by inducing highly localized pressure and temperature changes in the course of their action (Hogg and Freitas Jr. 2012).

Certain issues related to the manipulation and management must be resolved before the first actual trial is conducted. Most nanobots are assumed to be biocompatible, but it appears that ample attention has not been paid to their deployment and removal from the body after completion of the desired operation. Some nanobots are designed to degrade after they achieve their goals, but this makes them unstable to use in a real scenario. Also, the real-time imaging of most nanobots is not supported, which makes their manipulation and actuation even more challenging (Soto and Chrostowski 2018). The changes directly influence other sensing mechanisms like motion-based sensing in velocities of the nanobot units, and especially in the case of bubble-propelled devices, the jet stream also disrupts the nano-environments of the sensing electrodes of the nanobots, resulting in an inaccurate diagnosis (Kong, Guan, and Pumera 2018). The production of stray fields and fluctuations may further contribute to the same (Saxena et al. 2015).

As is the case with all innovative technologies, some ethical issues are also related to nanobots. For example, certain anti-social elements and terrorist groups may put them to various unintended evil uses. These applications may range from simple ones like inflicting torture to complicated ones like spying. Notwithstanding all these issues, any technology is good or evil depending on the user.

CONCLUSION

Nanobots are certainly the next frontier in many fields like environmental remediation and materials science. They are of particular significance in the field of biomedicine, because they are highly specific and precise to use and have the potential to demonstrate a versatile range of applications. From simple ones like helical swimmers to more complex molecular assortments like DNA clam-bots, nanorobots can prove to be instrumental in targeted drug administration and diagnosis of diseases as well as their treatment, whether surgically or through other physical means. Properties like self-propulsion, penetration, target-specificity, and swarming make the use of nanobots supremely desirable in medicine and there are ample instances of the *in-vivo* demonstrations of these properties. However, these were only proof-of-concept demonstrations, and specific issues like toxicity and biocompatibility, actuation and manipulation, and fuel-based propulsion in actual scenarios are yet to be observed. Once that has been done, this technology can prove to be pivotal in revolutionizing healthcare and medicine. This technology can be put to good use in the diagnosis of diseases in initial stages, cellular or very minute non-invasive surgeries, targeted drug delivery, and other therapeutic purposes.

To achieve all these advantages, we must address the challenges related to toxicity, fueling and powering, and synchronization at the earliest. Once that is done, this technology would undoubtedly prove to be highly advantageous over traditional biomedical practices. It will increase the efficacy of treatments and, subsequently, the life expectancy of patients. However, there are some ethical issues related to this technology, which make it a little unsafe when in the wrong hands, but that is dependent on the one who wields it.

REFERENCES

Abbott, Jake J., Kathrin E. Peyer, Marco Cosentino Lagomarsino, Li Zhang, Lixin Dong, Ioannis K. Kaliakatsos, and Bradley J. Nelson. 2009. "How Should Microrobots Swim?" *International Journal of Robotics Research* 28 (11–12): 1434–47. doi: 10.1177/0278364909341658.

Abdelmohsen, Loai K.E.A., Marlies Nijemeisland, Gajanan M. Pawar, Geert Jan A. Janssen, Roeland J.M. Nolte, Jan C.M. Van Hest, and Daniela A. Wilson. 2016. "Dynamic Loading and Unloading of Proteins in Polymeric Stomatocytes: Formation of an Enzyme-Loaded Supramolecular Nanomotor." *ACS Nano* 10 (2): 2652–60. doi: 10.1021/acsnano.5b07689.

Agrahari, Vibhuti, Vivek Agrahari, Ming-li Chou, Chew Ho Chew, James Noll, and Thierry Burnouf. 2020. "Intelligent Micro-/Nanorobots as Drug and Cell Carrier Devices for Biomedical Therapeutic Advancement: Promising Development Opportunities and Translational Challenges." *Biomaterials*. doi: 10.1016/j.biomaterials.2020.120163.

Ahmad, Md. Aquil, Ashar Kamal, Farhan Ashraf, and Abdul Fahed Ansari. 2014. "A Review on Current Scenario in the Field of Nanorobotics." *International Journal of Engineering Sciences & Research Technology* 3 (June): 578–84.

Akin, Demir, Jennifer Sturgis, Kathy Ragheb, Debby Sherman, Kristin Burkholder, J. Paul Robinson, Arun K. Bhunia, Sulma Mohammed, and Rashid Bashir. 2007. "Bacteria-Mediated Delivery of Nanoparticles and Cargo into Cells." *Nature Nanotechnology* 2 (7): 441–49. doi: 10.1038/nnano.2007.149.

Al-Hudhud, Ghada. 2012. "On Swarming Medical Nanorobots." *International Journal of Bio-Science and Bio-Technology* 4 (1): 75–90.

Ali, Jamel, U. Kei Cheang, James D. Martindale, Mehdi Jabbarzadeh, Henry C. Fu, and Min Jun Kim. 2017. "Bacteria-Inspired Nanorobots with Flagellar Polymorphic Transformations and Bundling." *Scientific Reports* 7 (1): 1–10. doi: 10.1038/s41598-017-14457-y.

Amendola, Valeria, Luigi Fabbrizzi, Carlo Mangano, and Piersandro Pallavicini. 2001. "Molecular Machines Based on Metal Ion Translocation." *Accounts of Chemical Research* 34 (6): 488–93. doi: 10.1021/ar010011c.

Amir, Yaniv, Eldad Ben-Ishay, Daniel Levner, Shmulik Ittah, Almogit Abu-Horowitz, and Ido Bachelet. 2014. "Universal Computing by DNA Origami Robots in a Living Animal." *Nature Nanotechnology* 9 (5): 353–57. doi: 10.1038/nnano.2014.58.

de Ávila, Berta Esteban Fernández, Pavimol Angsantikul, Doris E. Ramírez-Herrera, Fernando Soto, Hazhir Teymourian, Diana Dehaini, Yijie Chen, Liangfang Zhang, and Joseph Wang. 2018. "Hybrid Biomembrane-Functionalized Nanorobots for Concurrent Removal of Pathogenic Bacteria and Toxins." *Science Robotics* 3 (18): 17–22. doi.org/10.1126/scirobotics.aat0485.

AZoNano. 2017. "Protein-Based Nanotechnology." 2017. https://www.azonano.com/article.aspx?/ArticleID=4658.

Balzani, Vincenzo, Marcos Gómez-López, and J. Fraser Stoddart. 1998. "Molecular Machines." *Accounts of Chemical Research* 31 (7): 405–14. doi: 10.1021/ar970340y.

Barbash, Gabriel I., and Sherry A. Glied. 2010. "New Technology and Health Care Costs – The Case of Robot-Assisted Surgery." *New England Journal of Medicine* 363 (8): 701–04. doi: 10.1056/NEJMp1006602.

Bath, Jonathan, and Andrew J. Turberfield. 2007. "DNA Nanomachines." *Nature Nanotechnology* 2 (5): 275–84. doi: 10.1038/nnano.2007.104.

Bell, Dominik J., Stefan Leutenegger, K. M. Hammar, Lixin X. Dong, and Bradley J. Nelson. 2007. "Flagella-Like Propulsion for Microrobots Using a Nanocoil and a Rotating Electromagnetic Field." In *Proceedings – IEEE International Conference on Robotics and Automation*, 1128–33. doi: 10.1109/ROBOT.2007.363136.

Bogue, Robert. 2010. "Microrobots and Nanorobots: A Review of Recent Developments." *Industrial Robot* 37 (4): 341–46. doi: 10.1108/01439911011044796.

Bumb, Swapnil S., Dara J. Bhaskar, and Himanshu Punia. 2013. "Nanorobots & Challenges Faced by Nanodentistry." *Guident* 6 (September): 8–11.

Bunea, Ada Ioana, Ileana Alexandra Pavel, Sorin David, and Szilveszter Gáspár. 2015. "Sensing Based on the Motion of Enzyme-Modified Nanorods." *Biosensors and Bioelectronics* 67: 42–48. doi: 10.1016/j.bios.2014.05.062.

Büther, Florian, Florian-Lennert Lau, Marc Stelzner, and Sebastian Ebers. 2017. "A Formal Definition for Nanorobots and Nanonetworks." In *Springer International Publishing AG 2017*, edited by Olga Galinina, Sergey Andreev, Sergey Balandin, and Yevgeni Koucheryavy, vol. 10531, pp. 214–26. Lecture Notes in Computer Science. Cham: Springer International Publishing. doi: 10.1007/978-3-319-67380-6_20.

Carlsen, Rika Wright, Matthew R. Edwards, Jiang Zhuang, Cecile Pacoret, and Metin Sitti. 2014. "Magnetic Steering Control of Multi-Cellular Bio-Hybrid Microswimmers." *Lab on a Chip* 14 (19): 3850–59. doi: 10.1039/c4lc00707g.

Cavalcanti, Adriano, Tad Hogg, and Bijan Shirinzadeh. 2006. "Nanorobotics System Simulation in 3D Workspaces with Low Reynolds Number." In *2006 IEEE International Symposium on MicroNanoMechanical and Human Science*, 1–6. doi: 10.1109/MHS.2006.320269.

Cavalcanti, Adriano, Bijan Shirinzadeh, Robert A. Freitas, and Tad Hogg. 2008. "Nanorobot Architecture for Medical Target Identification." *Nanotechnology* 19 (1). doi: 10.1088/0957-4484/19/01/015103.

Chen, Chuanrui, Xiaocong Chang, Pavimol Angsantikul, Jinxing Li, Berta Esteban-Fernández de Ávila, Emil Karshalev, Wenjuan Liu, et al. 2018. "Chemotactic Guidance of Synthetic Organic/Inorganic Payloads Functionalized Sperm Micromotors." *Advanced Biosystems* 2 (1): 1700160. doi: 10.1002/adbi.201700160.

Chen, Chuanrui, Fangzhi Mou, Leilei Xu, Shaofei Wang, Jianguo Guan, Zunpeng Feng, Quanwei Wang, et al. 2017. "Light-Steered Isotropic Semiconductor Micromotors." *Advanced Materials* 29 (3). doi: 10.1002/adma.201603374.

Chen, Xiang Zhong, Marcus Hoop, Fajer Mushtaq, Erdem Siringil, Chengzhi Hu, Bradley J. Nelson, and Salvador Pané. 2017. "Recent Developments in Magnetically Driven Micro- and Nanorobots." *Applied Materials Today* 9: 37–48. doi: 10.1016/j.apmt.2017.04.006.

Dahmen, Christian, Tim Wortmann, and Sergej Fatikow. 2012. "Actuation and Tracking of Ferromagnetic Objects Using MRI." *International Journal of Optomechatronics* 6 (4): 321–35. doi: 10.1080/15599612.2012.721866.

Dai, Baohu, Jizhuang Wang, Ze Xiong, Xiaojun Zhan, Wei Dai, Chien Cheng Li, Shien Ping Feng, and Jinyao Tang. 2016. "Programmable Artificial Phototactic Microswimmer." *Nature Nanotechnology* 11 (12): 1087–92. doi: 10.1038/nnano.2016.187.

Devasena Umai, R., P. Brindha Devi, and R. Thiruchelvi. 2018. "A Review on DNA Nanobots – A New Technique for Cancer Treatment." *Asian Journal of Pharmaceutical and Clinical Research* 11 (6): 61–64. doi: 10.22159/ajpcr.2018.v11i6.25015.

Dey, Krishna Kanti, and Ayusman Sen. 2017. "Chemically Propelled Molecules and Machines." *Journal of the American Chemical Society* 139 (23): 7666–76. doi: 10.1021/jacs.7b02347.

Dey, Krishna Kanti, Xi Zhao, Benjamin M. Tansi, Wilfredo J. Méndez-Ortiz, Ubaldo M. Córdova-Figueroa, Ramin Golestanian, and Ayusman Sen. 2015. "Micromotors Powered by Enzyme Catalysis." *Nano Letters* 15 (12): 8311–15. doi: 10.1021/acs.nanolett.5b03935.

Dolev, Shlomi, Ram Prasadh Narayanan, and Michael Rosenblit. 2019. "Design of Nanorobots for Exposing Cancer Cells." *Nanotechnology* 30: 31. doi: 10.1088/1361-6528/ab1770.

Douglas, Shawn M., Ido Bachelet, and George M. Church. 2012. "A Logic-Gated Nanorobot for Targeted Transport of Molecular Payloads." *Science* 335 (6070): 831–34. doi: 10.1126/science.1214081.

Dressler, Falko, and Frank Kargl. 2012. "Towards Security in Nano-Communication: Challenges and Opportunities." *Nano Communication Networks* 3 (3): 151–60. doi: 10.1016/j.nancom.2012.08.001.

Elbaz, Johann, and Itamar Willner. 2012. "DNA Origami: Nanorobots Grab Cellular Control." *Nature Materials* 11 (4): 276–77. doi: 10.1038/nmat3287.

Feynman, Richard P. 1960. "There's Plenty of Room at the Bottom: The Nanometer Sizescale." *Caltech's Engineering and Science*, February: 1–11. http://www.zyvex.com/nanotech/feynman.html.

Fournier-Bidoz, Sébastien, André C. Arsenault, Ian Manners, and Geoffrey A. Ozin. 2005. "Synthetic Self-Propelled Nanorotors." *Chemical Communications*, 4: 441–43. doi: 10.1039/b414896g.

Gao, Wei, Xiaomiao Feng, Allen Pei, Christopher R. Kane, Ryan Tam, Camille Hennessy, and Joseph Wang. 2014. "Bioinspired Helical Microswimmers Based on Vascular Plants." *Nano Letters* 14 (1): 305–10. doi: 10.1021/nl404044d.

Gao, Wei, Allen Pei, and Joseph Wang. 2012. "Water-Driven Micromotors." *ACS Nano* 6 (9): 8432–38. doi: 10.1021/nn303309z.

Gao, Wei, Sirilak Sattayasamitsathit, Jahir Orozco, and Joseph Wang. 2011. "Highly Efficient Catalytic Microengines: Template Electrosynthesis of Polyaniline/Platinum Microtubes." *Journal of the American Chemical Society* 133 (31): 11862–64. doi: 10.1021/ja203773g.

Gao, Wei, and Joseph Wang. 2014. "Synthetic Micro/Nanomotors in Drug Delivery." *Nanoscale* 6 (18): 10486–94. doi: 10.1039/c4nr03124e.

Guix, Maria, Carmen C. Mayorga-Martinez, and Arben Merkoçi. 2014. "Nano/Micromotors in (Bio)Chemical Science Applications." *Chemical Reviews* 114 (12): 6285–322. doi: 10.1021/cr400273r.

Harada, Akira. 2001. "Cyclodextrin-Based Molecular Machines." *Accounts of Chemical Research* 34 (6): 456–64. doi: 10.1021/ar0001741.

Hogg, Tad, and Robert A. Freitas Jr. 2012. "Acoustic Communication for Medical Nanorobots." *Nano Communication Networks* 3 (2): 83–102. doi: 10.1016/j.nancom.2012.02.002.

Ibele, Michael E., Paul E. Lammert, Vincent H. Crespi, and Ayusman Sen. 2010. "Emergent, Collective Oscillations of Self-Mobile Particles and Patterned Surfaces under Redox Conditions." *ACS Nano* 4 (8): 4845–51. doi: 10.1021/nn101289p.

Ibele, Michael, Thomas E. Mallouk, and Ayusman Sen. 2009. "Schooling Behavior of Light-Powered Autonomous Micromotors in Water." *Angewandte Chemie International Edition* 48 (18): 3308–12. doi: 10.1002/anie.200804704.

Jarosz, Paul, Christopher Schauerman, Jack Alvarenga, Brian Moses, Thomas Mastrangelo, Ryne Raffaelle, Richard Ridgley, and Brian Landi. 2011. "Carbon Nanotube Wires and Cables: Near-Term Applications and Future Perspectives." *Nanoscale* 3 (11): 4542–53. doi: 10.1039/C1NR10814J.

Katuri, Jaideep, Xing Ma, Morgan M. Stanton, and Samuel Sánchez. 2017. "Designing Micro- and Nanoswimmers for Specific Applications." *Accounts of Chemical Research* 50 (1): 2–11. doi: 10.1021/acs.accounts.6b00386.

Khalil, Islam S. M., Veronika Magdanz, Samuel Sánchez, Oliver G. Schmidt, and Sarthak Misra. 2014. "Biocompatible, Accurate, and Fully Autonomous: A Sperm-Driven Micro-Bio-Robot." *Journal of Micro-Bio Robotics* 9 (3): 79–86. doi: 10.1007/s12213-014-0077-9.

Kim, Sangwon, Seungmin Lee, Jeonghun Lee, Bradley J. Nelson, Li Zhang, and Hongsoo Choi. 2016. "Fabrication and Manipulation of Ciliary Microrobots with Non-Reciprocal Magnetic Actuation." *Scientific Reports* 6 (March): 1–9. doi: 10.1038/srep30713.

Kong, Lei, Jianguo Guan, and Martin Pumera. 2018. "Micro- and Nanorobots Based Sensing and Biosensing."*Current Opinion in Electrochemistry* 10: 174–82. doi: 10.1016/j.coelec.2018.06.004.

Kostarelos, Kostas. 2010. "Editorial: Nanorobots for Medicine: How Close Are We?" *Nanomedicine* 5 (3): 341–42. doi: 10.2217/nnm.10.19.

Kotesa, Rahul S., Jitendra S. Rathore, and Nithya Nand Sharma. 2013. "Tapered Flagellated Nanoswimmer: Comparison of Helical Wave and Planar Wave Propulsion." *BioNanoScience* 3 (4): 343–47. doi: 10.1007/s12668-013-0105-6.

Kwon, Diana. 2018. "Researchers Develop Sperm-Robot Hybrids to Deliver Drugs, Assist Fertilization." *The Scientist*, 2018. https://www.the-scientist.com/notebook/researchers-develop-sperm-robot-hybrids-to-deliver-drugs-assist-fertilization-29858.

Lanfranco, Anthony R., Andres E. Castellanos, Jaydev P. Desai, and William C. Meyers. 2004. "Robotic Surgery: A Current Perspective." *Annals of Surgery* 239 (1): 14–21. doi: 10.1097/01.sla.0000103020.19595.7d.

Laocharoensuk, Rawiwan, Jared Burdick, and Joseph Wang. 2008. "Carbon-Nanotube-Induced Acceleration of Catalytic Nanomotors." *ACS Nano* 2 (5): 1069–75. doi: 10.1021/nn800154g.

Li, Jinxing, Pavimol Angsantikul, Wenjuan Liu, Berta Esteban-Fernández de Ávila, Xiaocong Chang, Elodie Sandraz, Yuyan Liang, et al. 2018. "Biomimetic Platelet-Camouflaged Nanorobots for Binding and Isolation of Biological Threats." *Advanced Materials* 30 (2): 1–8. doi: 10.1002/adma.201704800.

Li, Jinxing, Berta Esteban-Fernández de Ávila, Wei Gao, Liangfang Zhang, and Joseph Wang. 2019. "Micro/Nanorobots for Biomedicine: Delivery, Surgery, Sensing, and Detoxification." *Science Robotics* 176 (1): 1570–73. doi: 10.1038/s41395-018-0061-4.

Li, Jinxing, Isaac Rozen, and Joseph Wang. 2016. "Rocket Science at the Nanoscale." *ACS Nano* 10 (6): 5619–34. doi: 10.1021/acsnano.6b02518.

Li, Suping, Qiao Jiang, Shaoli Liu, Yinlong Zhang, Yanhua Tian, Chen Song, Jing Wang, et al. 2018. "A DNA Nanorobot Functions as a Cancer Therapeutic in Response to a Molecular Trigger In Vivo." *Nature Biotechnology* 36 (3): 258–64. doi: 10.1038/nbt.4071.

Li, Tianlong, Xiaocong Chang, Zhiguang Wu, Jinxing Li, Guangbin Shao, Xinghong Deng, Jianbin Qiu, et al. 2017. "Autonomous Collision-Free Navigation of Microvehicles in Complex and Dynamically Changing Environments." *ACS Nano* 11 (9): 9268–75. doi: 10.1021/acsnano.7b04525.

Lin, Xiankun, Zhiguang Wu, Yingjie Wu, Mingjun Xuan, and Qiang He. 2016. "Self-Propelled Micro-/Nanomotors Based on Controlled Assembled Architectures." *Advanced Materials* 28 (6): 1060–72. doi: 10.1002/adma.201502583.

Liu, Jian-Qin, and Tadashi Nakano. 2012. "Principles and Methods for Nanomechatronics: Signaling, Structure, and Functions Toward Nanorobots." *IEEE Transactions on Systems, Man, and Cybernetics, Part C (Applications and Reviews)* 42 (3): 357–66. doi: 10.1109/TSMCC.2011.2119481.

Liu, Ran, and Ayusman Sen. 2011. "Autonomous Nanomotor Based on Copper-Platinum Segmented Nanobattery." *Journal of the American Chemical Society* 133 (50): 20064–67. doi: 10.1021/ja2082735.

Loukanov, Alexandre, Hristo Gagov, and Seiichiro Nakabayashi. 2020. "Artificial Nanomachines and Nanorobotics." In, 515–32. doi: 10.1201/9781003027010-14.

Loukanov, Alexandre, Ryota Sekiya, Midori Yoshikawa, Naritaka Kobayashi, Yuji Moriyasu, and Seiichiro Nakabayashi. 2016. "Photosensitizer-Conjugated Ultrasmall Carbon Nanodots as Multifunctional Fluorescent Probes for Bioimaging." *The Journal of Physical Chemistry C* 120 (29): 15867–74. doi: 10.1021/acs.jpcc.5b11721.

Ma, Xing, Anita Jannasch, Urban Raphael Albrecht, Kersten Hahn, Albert Miguel-López, Erik Schäffer, and Samuel Sánchez. 2015. "Enzyme-Powered Hollow Mesoporous Janus Nanomotors." *Nano Letters* 15 (10): 7043–50. doi: 10.1021/acs.nanolett.5b03100.

Ma, Xing, and Samuel Sánchez. 2017. "Self-Propelling Micro-Nanorobots: Challenges and Future Perspectives in Nanomedicine." *Nanomedicine* 12 (12): 1363–67.

Ma, Xing, Xu Wang, Kersten Hahn, and Samuel Sánchez. 2016. "Motion Control of Urea-Powered Biocompatible Hollow Microcapsules." *ACS Nano* 10 (3): 3597–605. doi: 10.1021/acsnano.5b08067.

Magdanz, Veronika, Maria Guix, Franziska Hebenstreit, and Oliver G. Schmidt. 2016. "Dynamic Polymeric Microtubes for the Remote-Controlled Capture, Guidance, and Release of Sperm Cells." *Advanced Materials* 28 (21): 4084–89. doi: 10.1002/adma.201505487.

Magdanz, Veronika, Mariana Medina-Sánchez, Yan Chen, Maria Guix, and Oliver G. Schmidt. 2015. "How to Improve Spermbot Performance." *Advanced Functional Materials* 25 (18): 2763–70. doi: 10.1002/adfm.201500015.

Magdanz, Veronika, Georgi Stoychev, Leonid Ionov, Samuel Sánchez, and Oliver G. Schmidt. 2014. "Stimuli-Responsive Microjets with Reconfigurable Shape." *Angewandte Chemie* 126 (10): 2711–15. doi: 10.1002/ange.201308610.

Mahadevan, L., and P. Matsudaira. 2000. "Motility Powered by Supramolecular Springs and Ratchets." *Science* 288 (5463): 95–99. doi: 10.1126/science.288.5463.95.

Maheswari, Raja, S. Sheeba Rani, V. Gomathy, and P. Sharmila. 2018. "Cancer Detecting Nanobot Using Positron Emission Tomography." *Procedia Computer Science* 133: 315–22. doi: 10.1016/j.procs.2018.07.039.

Malewar, Amit. 2016. "Actuating Nano-Transducers the World's Tiniest Engine." *Tech Explorist*. May 3, 2016. https://www.techexplorist.com/actuating-nano-transducers/2607/.

Mallouk, Thomas E., and Ayusman Sen. 2009. "Powering Nanorobots." *Scientific American* 300 (5): 72–77. http://www.jstor.org/stable/26001346.

Manesh, Kalayil Manian, Shankar Balasubramanian, and Joseph Wang. 2010. "Nanomotor-Based 'writing' of Surface Microstructures." *Chemical Communications* 46 (31): 5704–06. doi: 10.1039/c0cc00178c.

Manjunath, Apoorva, and Vijay Kishore. 2014. "The Promising Future in Medicine: Nanorobots." *Biomedical Science and Engineering* 2 (2): 42–47. doi: 10.12691/bse-2-2-3.

Martel, Sylvain. 2011. "Flagellated Bacterial Nanorobots for Medical Interventions in the Human Body." *Surgical Robotics: Systems Applications and Visions*, 397–416. doi: 10.1007/978-1-4419-1126-1.

Martins, Nuno R. B., Wolfram Erlhagen, and Robert A. Freitas. 2012. "Non-Destructive Whole-Brain Monitoring Using Nanorobots: Neural Electrical Data Rate Requirements." *International Journal of Machine Consciousness* 4 (1): 109–40. doi: 10.1142/S1793843012400069.

Mavroidis, Constantinos, and Antoine Ferreira. 2013. "Nanorobotics: Past, Present, and Future BT – Nanorobotics: Current Approaches and Techniques." In, edited by Constantinos Mavroidis and Antoine Ferreira, 3–27. New York, NY: Springer. doi: 10.1007/978-1-4614-2119-1_1.

Mazumder, Sujayita, Roy Biswas, and Sutapa Biswas Majee. 2020. "Applications of Nanorobots in Medical Techniques." *International Journal of Pharmaceutical Sciences and Research* 11 (7): 3150. doi: 10.13040/IJPSR.0975-8232.11(7).3150-59.

Medina-Sánchez, Mariana, Lukas Schwarz, Anne K. Meyer, Franziska Hebenstreit, and Oliver G. Schmidt. 2016. "Cellular Cargo Delivery: Toward Assisted Fertilization by Sperm-Carrying Micromotors." *Nano Letters* 16 (1): 555–61. doi: 10.1021/acs.nanolett.5b04221.

Mertz, Leslie. 2018. "Tiny Conveyance: Micro- and Nanorobots Prepare to Advance Medicine." *IEEE Pulse* 9 (1): 19–23.

Mitthra, Suresh, Arumugam Karthick, Balasubramaniam Anuradha, Radhakrishnan Mensudar, Kalyani Ramkumar Sadhana, and Gurubaran Nidhya Varshini. 2016. "Nanorobots – A Small Wonder." *Biosciences, Biotechnology Research Asia* 13 (4): 2131–34. doi: 10.13005/bbra/2374.

Mou, Fangzhi, Chuanrui Chen, Huiru Ma, Yixia Yin, Qingzhi Wu, and Jianguo Guan. 2013. "Self-Propelled Micromotors Driven by the Magnesium-Water Reaction and Their Hemolytic Properties." *Angewandte Chemie - International Edition* 52 (28): 7208–12. doi: 10.1002/anie.201300913.

Nelson, Bradley J., and Kathrin E. Peyer. 2014. "Micro- and Nanorobots Swimming in Heterogeneous Liquids." *ACS Nano* 8 (9): 8718–24. doi: 10.1021/nn504295z.

Nelson, Bryn. 2008. "Scientists Look to Sperm to Power Nanobots – Technology & Science – Innovation." *Frontiers on NBC NEWS*. February 1, 2008. http://www.nbcnews.com/id/22333518/ns/technology_and_science-innovation/t/scientists-look-sperm-power-nanobots/#.Xyb5iygza00.

Oiwa, K. 2003. "Protein Motors: Their Mechanical Properties and Application to Nanometer-Scale Devices." *Materials Science Forum* 426–4: 2339–44. https://www.cheric.org/research/tech/periodicals/view.php?seq=1254733.

Padovani, Gislaine C., Victor P. Feitosa, Salvatore Sauro, Franklin R. Tay, Gabriela Durán, Amauri J. Paula, and Nelson Durán. 2015. "Advances in Dental Materials through Nanotechnology: Facts, Perspectives and Toxicological Aspects." *Trends in Biotechnology* 33 (11): 621–36. doi: 10.1016/j.tibtech.2015.09.005.

Pané, Salvador, Josep Puigmartí-Luis, Christos Bergeles, Xiang-Zhong Chen, Eva Pellicer, Jordi Sort, Vanda Počepcová, Antoine Ferreira, and Bradley J. Nelson. 2019. "Imaging Technologies for Biomedical Micro- and Nanoswimmers." *Advanced Materials Technologies* 4 (4): 1800575. doi: 10.1002/admt.201800575.

Patil, Lalita Balasaheb, Swapnil S. Patil, Manoj M. Nitalikar, Chandrakant S. Magdum, and Shrinivas K. Mohite. 2016. "A Review On-Novel Approaches in Nanorobotics." *Asian Journal of Pharmaceutical Research* 6 (4): 217–24. doi: 10.5958/2231-5691.2016.00030.7.

Pavlick, Ryan A., Samudra Sengupta, Timothy McFadden, Hua Zhang, and Ayusman Sen. 2011. "A Polymerization-Powered Motor." *Angewandte Chemie International Edition* 50 (40): 9374–77. doi: 10.1002/anie.201103565.

Paxton, Walter F., Kevin C. Kistler, Christine C. Olmeda, Ayusman Sen, Sarah K. St. Angelo, Yanyan Cao, Thomas E. Mallouk, Paul E. Lammert, and Vincent H. Crespi. 2004. "Catalytic Nanomotors: Autonomous Movement of Striped Nanorods." *Journal of the American Chemical Society* 126 (41): 13424–31. doi: 10.1021/ja047697z.

Qiu, Famin, and Bradley J. Nelson. 2015. "Magnetic Helical Micro- and Nanorobots: Toward Their Biomedical Applications." *Engineering* 1 (1): 21–26. doi: 10.15302/J-ENG-2015005.

Requicha, Aristides A. G. 2003. "Nanorobots, NEMS, and Nanoassembly." *Proceedings of the IEEE* 91 (11): 1922–33. doi: 10.1109/JPROC.2003.818333.

Satir, Peter. 1999. "The Cilium as a Biological Nano-Machine." *The FASEB Journal* 13 (9002): 235–37. doi: 10.1096/fasebj.13.9002.s235.

Saxena, Shweta, B. J. Pramod, B. C. Dayananda, and Kanneboyina Nagaraju. 2015. "Design, Architecture and Application of Nanorobotics in Oncology." *Indian Journal of Cancer* 52 (2): 236–41. doi: 10.4103/0019-509X.175805.

Schuerle, Simone, Salvador Pané, Eva Pellicer, Jordi Sort, Maria D. Baró, and Bradley J. Nelson. 2012. "Helical and Tubular Lipid Microstructures That Are Electroless-Coated with CoNiReP for Wireless Magnetic Manipulation." *Small* 8 (10): 1498–502. doi: 10.1002/smll.201101821.

Senanayake, Arosha, R. G. Sirisinghe, and Phang Shih Mun. 2007. "Nanorobot: Modelling and Simulation." In *International Conference on Control, Instrumentation and Mechatronics Engineering*, 453–58. Johor Bahru, Johor, Malaysia.

Sengupta, Samudra, Michael E. Ibele, and Ayusman Sen. 2012. "Fantastic Voyage: Designing Self-Powered Nanorobots." *Angewandte Chemie – International Edition* 51 (34): 8434–45. doi: 10.1002/anie.201202044.

Servick, Kelly. 2016. "Video: Motorized 'Spermbot' Helps Sperm Reach Egg." *Science*, January. doi: 10.1126/science.aae0224.

Sim, Seunghyun, and Takuzo Aida. 2017. "Swallowing a Surgeon: Toward Clinical Nanorobots." *Accounts of Chemical Research* 50 (3): 492–97. doi: 10.1021/acs.accounts.6b00495.

Sivasankar, Mahalakshmi, and Raj B. Durairaj. 2012. "Brief Review on Nano Robots in Bio Medical Applications." *Advances in Robotics & Automation* 1 (1): 1–4. doi: 10.4172/2168-9695.1000101.

Soong, Ricky K., George D. Bachand, Hercules P. Neves, Anatoli G. Olkhovets, Harold G. Craighead, and Carlo D. Montemagno. 2000. "Powering an Inorganic Nanodevice with a Biomolecular Motor." *Science* 290 (5496): 1555–58. doi: 10.1126/science.290.5496.1555.

Soto, Fernando, and Robert Chrostowski. 2018. "Frontiers of Medical Micro/Nanorobotics: In Vivo Applications and Commercialization Perspectives Toward Clinical Uses." *Frontiers in Bioengineering and Biotechnology* 6 (November): 1–12. doi: 10.3389/fbioe.2018.00170.

Spendlove, Tom. 2014. "Surgical Nanorobots – A Moonshot Project." *Engineering.Com.* May 12, 2014. https://www.engineering.com/DesignSoftware/DesignSoftwareArticles/ArticleID/7583/Surgical-Nanorobots--A-Moonshot-Project.aspx.

Srivastava, Sarvesh Kumar, Mariana Medina-Sánchez, Britta Koch, and Oliver G. Schmidt. 2016. "Medibots: Dual-Action Biogenic Microdaggers for Single-Cell Surgery and Drug Release." *Advanced Materials* 28 (5): 832–37. doi: 10.1002/adma.201504327.

Strong, Michael. 2004. "Protein Nano-machines." *PLoS Biology* 2 (3): 305–06. doi: 10.1371/journal.pbio.0020073.

Torney, François, Brian G. Trewyn, Victor S.-Y. Lin, and Kan Wang. 2007. "Mesoporous Silica Nanoparticles Deliver DNA and Chemicals into Plants." *Nature Nanotechnology* 2 (5): 295–300. doi: 10.1038/nnano.2007.108.

Tørring, Thomas, Niels V. Voigt, Jeanette Nangreave, Hao Yan, and Kurt V. Gothelf. 2011. "DNA Origami: A Quantum Leap for Self-Assembly of Complex Structures." *Chemical Society Reviews* 40 (12): 5621–928. doi: 10.1039/c1cs15057j.

Tyreman, Matthew J. A., and Justin E. Molloy. 2003. "Molecular Motors: Nature's Nanomachines." *IEE Proceedings – Nanobiotechnology* 150 (3): 95–102. doi: 10.1049/ip-nbt:20031172.

Ullrich, Franziska, Christos Bergeles, Juho Pokki, Olgac Ergeneman, Sandro Erni, George Chatzipirpiridis, Salvador Pané, Carsten Framme, and Bradley J. Nelson. 2013. "Mobility Experiments with Microrobots for Minimally Invasive Intraocular Surgery." *Investigative Ophthalmology & Visual Science* 54 (4): 2853–63. doi: 10.1167/iovs.13-11825.

Ummat, Ajay, Gaurav Sharma, Constantinos Mavroidis, and Anshu Dubey. 2016. "Robotics: State of the Art and Future Challenges." In *Tissue Engineering and Artificial Robots*, 309–54. CRC Press. doi: 10.1142/P542.

Vach, Peter J., Peter Fratzl, Stefan Klumpp, and Damien Faivre. 2015. "Fast Magnetic Micropropellers with Random Shapes." *Nano Letters* 15 (10): 7064–70. doi: 10.1021/acs.nanolett.5b03131.

Venkatesan, Mithra, and Bhuvaneshwari Jolad. 2010. "Nanorobots in Cancer Treatment." In *International Conference on 'Emerging Trends in Robotics and Communication Technologies'*, INTERACT-2010, 258–64. doi: 10.1109/INTERACT.2010.5706154.

Wang, Hong, and Martin Pumera. 2015. "Fabrication of Micro/Nanoscale Motors." *Chemical Reviews* 115 (16): 8704–35. doi: 10.1021/acs.chemrev.5b00047.

Wang, Hong, and Martin Pumera. 2018. "Micro/Nano-machines and Living Biosystems: From Simple Interactions to Microcyborgs." *Advanced Functional Materials* 28 (25): 1705421. doi: 10.1002/adfm.201705421.

Wang, Hong, Guanjia Zhao, and Martin Pumera. 2014. "Crucial Role of Surfactants in Bubble-Propelled Microengines." *Journal of Physical Chemistry C* 118 (10): 5268–74. doi: 10.1021/jp410003e.

Wang, Joseph. 2016. "Self-Propelled Affinity Biosensors: Moving the Receptor around the Sample." *Biosensors and Bioelectronics* 76: 234–42. doi: 10.1016/j.bios.2015.04.095.

Wen, Zhi-Bin, Xin Peng, Ze-Zhou Yang, Ying Zhuo, Ya-Qin Chai, Wen-Bin Liang, and Ruo Yuan. 2019. "A Dynamic 3D DNA Nanostructure Based on Silicon-Supported Lipid Bilayers: A Highly Efficient DNA Nano-machine for Rapid and Sensitive Sensing." *Chemical Communications* 55 (89): 13414–17. doi: 10.1039/C9CC07071K.

Whitesides, George M. 2001. "The Once and Future Nanomachine." *Scientific American* 285 (3): 70. doi: 10.1038/scientificamerican0901-78.

Wilson, Damien Jonas, M.D., 2018. "Nanorobotic Devices," 1–4. https://www.news-medical. net/health/Nanorobotic-Devices.aspx

Xuan, Mingjun, Zhiguang Wu, Jingxin Shao, Luru Dai, Tieyan Si, and Qiang He. 2016. "Near Infrared Light-Powered Janus Mesoporous Silica Nanoparticle Motors." *Journal of the American Chemical Society* 138 (20): 6492–97. doi: 10.1021/jacs.6b00902.

Zhang, Huigang, Xindi Yu, and Paul V. Braun. 2011. "Three-Dimensional Bicontinuous Ultrafast-Charge and Discharge Bulk Battery Electrodes." *Nature Nanotechnology* 6 (5): 277–81. doi: 10.1038/nnano.2011.38.

Zhang, Li, Jake J. Abbott, Lixin Dong, Kathrin E. Peyer, Bradley E. Kratochvil, Haixin Zhang, Christos Bergeles, and Bradley J. Nelson. 2009. "Characterizing the Swimming Properties of Artificial Bacterial Flagella." *Nano Letters* 9 (10): 3663–67. doi: 10.1021/ nl901869j.

Zhang, Li, Tristan Petit, Yang Lu, Bradley E. Kratochvil, Kathrin E. Peyer, Ryan Pei, Jun Lou, and Bradley J. Nelson. 2010. "Controlled Propulsion and Cargo Transport of Rotating Nickel Nanowires near a Patterned Solid Surface." *ACS Nano* 4 (10): 6228–34. doi: 10.1021/nn101861n.

Zhou, Yu-Jie, Yuan-Hui Wan, Cun-Peng Nie, Juan Zhang, Ting-Ting Chen, and Xia Chu. 2019. "Molecular Switching of a Self-Assembled 3D DNA Nano-Machine for Spatiotemporal pH Mapping in Living Cells." *Analytical Chemistry* 91 (16): 10366–70. doi: 10.1021/ acs.analchem.9b02514.

3 Communicable Diseases and COVID-19: A Complementary and Holistic Care with Robotic Renaissance

S. Jeelani
Sri Venkateshwaraa Dental College

CONTENTS

INTRODUCTION

Life is a blessing. Health is the blessing of life. Disease is one entity in science that causes an imbalance in health. *Health and disease are two important terms pertaining to life which respectively can be explained as an absolute physical and psychosocial wellness (not the mere absence of disease); deviation from body's normal function and is sometimes connected to the concept of illness.*[1,2] The destiny of life is unpredictable resulting from infinite known and unknown reasons including diseases. In a broader way, diseases can be categorized into communicable and non-communicable diseases.

COMMUNICABLE DISEASES

These diseases arise through transmission from an infected to a susceptible, either directly or indirectly.[3]

HISTORY OF INFECTIOUS DISEASES

Hippocrates, the father of Western medicine, is the pioneer in the history of infectious diseases.[4] Historically popular personalities like Pericles, Alexander, and romantic English poet John Keats have lost their lives due to infectious diseases. The mode of spread of infectious diseases has been quoted by Hippocrates and the germ theory was postulated by Fracastoro. History repeats and today it is COVID-19 that is threatening the entire world and is the unparalleled communicable disease.[5]

COVID-19 PANDEMIC AND PANDEMIC FEAR

PANDEMIC

It is a communicable disease spreading globally and rapidly affecting the susceptible with variable mortality and morbidity.[3]

Rational knowledge and power of intellect is one of the vital strengths of humans. On one side, researchers and humans are fighting against the virus, but the worst side of it is the fight of human emotion with this virus. Fear is one such emotion that is deeply engraved in every human today. Scientifically, fear can be described as an alarm to danger. In this context, it is prudent to connect to the scientific fact of alarm pheromones prominent among the wild world and today, researchers are associating it with the human race.

ALARM PHEROMONES AND SECOND-HAND STRESS

Pheromone is the term coined by Peter Karlson and Martin Lüscher in 1959. Alarm pheromones are chemical messengers that affect neurocircuits by olfaction and other senses and thus have an impact on human behavior and emotions. Amygdala is a structure in the brain, which is associated with emotions including fear.[6]

Experimental research was carried out with sweat samples of individuals with fear and the results are compared with those of normal individuals. Neuroimaging using fMRI (functional magnetic resonance imaging) revealed that neurobiological evidence existed for human alarm pheromone and as a result, the concept of second-hand stress evolved, which is equally a pandemic today and is equally infectious and contagious in juxtaposition to COVID-19.[7]

LEVELS OF COMMUNICABLE INFECTIONS

Exposure phase
Infection phase
Infectious disease phase
Outcome phase

EXPOSURE PHASE

Close contact of the susceptible host with the infectious agent without entry into the host's body cells.

INFECTION PHASE

Entry and multiplication of the infectious agent into the host's body without clinical manifestations of the disease.

INFECTIOUS DISEASE PHASE

The infected host manifests clinical manifestations of the disease.

OUTCOME PHASE

It is associated with recovery, disability, or death of the patient.[8]

TERMINOLOGIES AND DEFINITION

In the context of infection, it is important to realize and understand the different states of infection, which are associated with the significant terms "carrier", "contact", "contamination", "incubation period", "communicable period", "isolation", and "quarantine".

CARRIER

A *carrier* is one who harbors an infectious agent. A carrier may exist as an *asymptomatic carrier* or an *incubatory or convalescent carrier.*

CONTACT

A *contact* is one who is associated with an infectious agent.

INCUBATION PERIOD

It is that period between the contact and symptoms.

ISOLATION

It is the period of separation of the communicable period to prevent the spread of infection.

PERIOD OF COMMUNICABILITY/COMMUNICABLE PERIOD

It is the period during which there is a chance of transmission of infection.

QUARANTINE

It is the limitation of freedom of movement of the contacts during the period of communicability to prevent the spread of disease. It is classified as follows:

Absolute or complete quarantine: Complete limitation of freedom of movement during the communicable period.

Modified quarantine: Partial limitation of freedom of movement. It involves *personal surveillance* (recognition of infection) and *segregation* (separation of the infected from the susceptible).[3]

COVID-19 AND COMMUNICABLE DISEASES

Human creation is unique and the most superior of all creations. However, the threat to the human race has equally been present due to multiple factors from time immemorial. The world's history reminds us of such pandemic problems that were overcome with time and timely measures. Communicable diseases are one such potential threat, which cannot be ignored. Globally, WHO declares approximately 80 important communicable diseases. In the current scenario, no doubt COVID-19 is a pandemic threatening the entire world. Its origin has been speculated to be bats.[9]

STRUCTURE OF CORONAVIRUS

Spike like surface-level projections gives it a crown-like appearance under the electron microscope.[10]

TRANSMISSION OF THE VIRUS

Transmission is from infected droplets by means of either contact or inhalation. The incubation time is from approximately 2 days to 2 weeks.[11] Higher viral loads have been found in the nasal cavity.[12] Sodium hypochlorite and hydrogen peroxide serve as disinfectants against the surface contamination with droplets.[13] Post-natal transmission risk in neonates is suggested.[14]

CLINICAL FEATURES OF COVID-19

Cough, sore throat, rise in body temperature, headache, tiredness, muscle ache, and difficulty in breathing are common symptoms. In severe cases, pneumonia, respiratory failure, and death can occur.

CONVENTIONAL MANAGEMENT

Conventional management is basically to alleviate the symptoms. Social distancing in general and isolation of affected individuals are carried out to prevent transmission. In patients with breathing difficulties, oxygen supplementation and ventilator support are indicated. Antiviral drugs have been used, but specific treatment is researched.[15] Vaccine is under development.

COMPLEMENTARY CARE OF COVID-19

Complementary and holistic care in handling COVID-19 is adjunctively practiced to promote antibody production in the defensive role via adaptive immune system and per se innate immune system.[16–19] Three-fourths of the world population is adjunctively utilizing complementary and alternative medicines (CAMs) when allopathic medical management fails or is in dearth.[20]

Herbal sources of immune-boosting products such as curcumin obtained from turmeric, vitamins such as vitamin C and D, and zinc enhance the antibodies.[21–26] Innate and adaptive immune systems are modulated by vitamin D.[27] Research on the intravenous use of vitamin C and higher vitamin D_3 doses is explored.[28,29] Overall CAMs are under research as an immune defensive strategy against infectious diseases.[30]

GOVERNANCE MANAGEMENT OF PANDEMIC

International response to this coronavirus is a challenge of the century, especially to the governments to protect their people. Governance through an intellectual policy called One Health approach to pandemic outbreaks is noteworthy to mention. Effective One Health governance is a three-dimensional approach. The first dimension is detection denoted by surveillance; the second dimension is inter- and intrasector co-ordination; and the third dimension is a targeted focus on the high risk and susceptible ones.[31]

DIGITAL CARE AND COVID-19

The COVID-19 pandemic has evoked digital health care at peak levels from optional to essential. However, human touch expressing empathy and compassion is seldom felt as part of this digital divine. Physical presence, trust, and interpersonal connections are also lost in the digital world for some patients. Similarly, confidence and satisfaction among patients resulting from physical examination by doctors is a distant empathetic component in digital care. To face this challenge, advances in science have given birth to robots wherein technically embedded "web side manners" have been created to closely substitute empathetic human bedside manners.[32–39]

ROBOTIC CARE AND COMMUNICABLE DISEASES

Off late as COVID-19 pandemic is escalating, apart from the community, very pathetically health care workers are at greater risk, necessitating digital care and ultimately robotic care to support the medical fraternities has become essential which can operate from distance using remote control thus avoiding direct contact to the infectious environment. The role of a robot is multifaceted involving the roles of physician, nurse, surgeon, investigator, and occasionally even as a programmed companion for those in quarantine and ultimately serving as the need of the hour adjuvant sophisticated technological support, being guided by telemedicine as the crucial and most supportive critical caretakers without being susceptible to infection.

ROBOTIC RENAISSANCE

Karel Capek in 1920 coined the word *robot*, which means servant or worker in Czech. George Devol in 1954 designed the first programmable robot (UNIMATE). The Robotic Institute of America in 1979 has defined *robot*.

Apart from community spread, it is pathetic to note that despite stringent universal and special protective protocols, spread of viral infection in the hospital environment is affecting health workers at all levels starting from doctors, nurses, laboratory personnel, sanitary staff, and all groups of health workers. It is a bitter truth that treating and supporting health personnel are losing their lives to COVID. This merciless fact is pushing science to the best of its advances and it is here that the robotic renaissance is lending its timely support.

Robots have been used in multiple sectors for the past few years. However, their application in a hospital environment is expensive and needs the support of advanced technology. With COVID-19 reaching all over the world, it is the need of the hour that every country must invest in and utilize the robots for a noble human cause to evade the spread of infection, which is unpredictable and alarming because of the asymptomatic carrier states also being potential threats to valuable human life.[40-42]

VEEBOT – THE ROBOTIC INVESTIGATOR

Veebot is a sandwich advance in robotic science combining robotics and the imaging technology. It is used in the field of investigation. It is employed for drawing blood. Veebot mitigates the phlebotomist and serves as a binary boon. Veebots help insert intravenous catheters and draw blood from weak veins. The working principle of a Veebot is a bimodal technology utilizing infrared light sources for exploring a suitable vein and ultrasound to analyze the flow of blood. A Veebot is accurate and quick in its investigative ability. Its accuracy is approximately 83%.[43] With regards to COVID-19, the challenge lies in the collection of nasal swabs.

RP-7 – ROBOTIC PHYSICIAN

Every profession is connected to life. However, the field of medicine is an unparalleled noble profession. In today's scenario with COVID-19 pandemic on one end and COVID-19 pandemic fear on the other end, the selfless service provided by doctors and health professionals risking their lives is unmatched. However, to rescue and to reduce their burden, definitely robotic science is a massive backbone. RP-7 is a robotic doctor serving as round the clock physician bridging online duty doctors (without direct contact/without the need for travel) to patients in a crucial contagious situation such as COVID-19, thus serving as a noble scientific messenger connecting the physician and the patients.[44,45]

RIBA – ROBOTIC NURSE (ROBOT FOR INTERACTIVE BODY ASSISTANCE)

History reminds us of Florence Nightingale when we revere nurses. However, there are infinite unnoticed and less looked upon but most sacrificing and dedicated nurses who have stood by the doctors in selfless care of patients against severe communicable and contagious diseases. Even today, countless nurses have lost their lives in COVID wards. Arising as a silent surprise to this soulful profession is the interactive body assistance robots referred to as RIBA (robot for interactive body assistance) serving as a robot nurse. RIBA resembles a teddy bear made of urethane and weighs about 180 kg including the battery with tactile sensors. It lifts patients (up to 60 kg) with its flexible arms. It recognizes faces and voices. It also responds to vocal commands. Thus RIBA exhibits sympathetic and empathetic nursing care in all groups of patients including those with communicable diseases especially in a situation like COVID-19 where the medically compromised are the most prone, thus demanding the need for caretakers wherein no doubt RIBA justifies its role in being free from being infected by any modes.[46]

Bush Robot – Robotic Surgeon

Multiple surgeons are inevitably losing their precious lives amidst all possible protective measures in a selfless effort to save the lives of COVID patients. Encountering this most baffling situation is the *bush robot*. The bush robots possess trillions of nanoscale fingers resembling an animated bush. Their dexterity and swiftness by means of inbuilt software are excellent, which make them brilliant surgeons. Hans Moravec is the pioneer of the bush robots. The robots play a significant and sensible surgeon role in multiple pathologies and the future of contagious and communicable disease-related surgeries may be successfully and safely treated by the brilliant bush robot technology, when time paves a platform for robotics to be a scientific global support.[47]

Virtibot – A Robot in Forensic Imaging

It is a non-invasive 3D imaging technology using multi-slice computed tomography (MSCT) and magnetic resonance imaging (MRI) to explore the human body in the field of forensic science replacing conventional autopsy thereby decreasing the grief of the relatives of the deceased.[48,49]

Documentation of body surfaces and estimating the time since death are, respectively, performed by 3D surface scanning 3D/CAD photogrammetry and MRI spectroscopy.[50]

Virtibot bridges forensic, imaging, telematics, automatic, and digital science, and biomechanics.[51] In the current scenario of the pandemic, virtibot is a dynamic dimension in forensic science in the process of exploration of the human body virtually with robotic assistance.

Stevie Robot

Stevie is an interactive robot useful for quarantined people that communicates with them and definitely is the right companion for those with communicable diseases without the risk of infection transmission.

The Violet Robot

Violet is a navigator robot. By means of inbuilt sensors and automated light sources, it helps in the independent navigation of health workers in the infectious environment.

The Sterilization Robots

They are very useful in sterilization and disinfection of hospital wards and isolation rooms by using a pulsed xenon ultraviolet-C light (wavelengths between 200 and 280 nm) to wipe out pathogens, preventing hospital-acquired infections. Ultraviolet light causes DNA either to change shape or to act like molecular scissors cutting the genetic material in pathogens especially viruses.

Drones

Drones are flying robots useful in identifying those who are not wearing masks in public spaces, spraying disinfectant in public spaces, and identifying people with elevated body temperatures using thermal sensing.

Transport and Delivery Robots

Robots have been employed in food delivery and drug delivery to people in isolation, transport of drugs to hospitals, collecting patient samples, and automating lab tests.

HOLISTIC HERBAL CARE

Herbal medicine has been in practice since the dawn of history. Madagascar's 'Covid-Organics' (a plant-derived from Artemisia), which is anti-malarial, is researched for the treatment of COVID-19. Awareness, multidisciplinary research, legal compliance by government, policies to grow, protect, and utilize herbal medicine, investigating plant-based environmental conditions, and required economy to promote industries for processing are among the few vital measures to promote herbal care as a holistic complementary aid in communicable diseases.[52-58]

CONCLUSION

"Silent infection is the biggest potential threat & alarming scenario regarding COVID-19". "At this time, we really need to ensure that we have a global orchestrated sustainable approach to holistic and complementary care including robotics research. Everyone is afraid of the consequence of error. But the greatest error is not to move. The greatest error is to be paralyzed by the fear of failure".[59] It is the utmost responsibility of humans to work hard with unity and dedication to save the world and all its creations by virtue of their blessed rational knowledge and intellect in a selfless and altruistic attitude with loyalty, faithfulness, and gratitude to the Creator.

ACKNOWLEDGMENTS

I want to express my profound gratitude to Almighty, family, teachers, and all good souls in the contribution of this chapter to generations of today and future.

I sincerely acknowledge and thank the Publishers for giving me the platform to share my work expressing my salutes to all concerned with the care of patients with communicable diseases and COVID-19.

REFERENCES

1. Sartorius N. 2006. The meanings of health and its promotion. *Croat Med J.* 47(4):662–664.
2. Kenneth M.B. 2000. Disease, illness, sickness, health, healing and wholeness: exploring some elusive concepts. *J Med Ethics Med Humanities* 26:9–17.

3. David L.H. 2016. *Explanation of Terms. Control of Communicable Diseases Manual.* Washington, DC: APHA Press.

4. Pappas G., Kiriaze I.J., Falagas M.E. 2008. Insights into infectious disease in the era of Hippocrates. *Int J Inf Dis.* 12(3):347–350.

5. Burke A.C. 2004. Historical aspects of infectious diseases. Part I. *Infect Dis Clin North Am.* 18(1): xi–xv.

6. Brennan P.A. 2010. *The Neurobiology of Olfaction. Pheromones and Mammalian Behavior.* Boca Raton, FL: Taylor and Francis Group, LLC.

7. Mujica-Parodi L.R., Helmut H.S., Frederick B., et al. 2008. Second-hand stress: neuro-biological evidence for a human alarm pheromone. *Nature Proceedings.* doi: 10.1038/npre.2008.2561.1.

8. Bhopal R.S. 2008. *Interrelated Concepts in the Epidemiology of Disease: Natural History, Spectrum, Iceberg, Population Patterns, and Screening. Concepts of Epidemiology: Integrating the Ideas, Theories, Principles, and Methods of Epidemiology,* 2nd ed. Oxford: Oxford University Press.

9. Singhal T. 2020. A review of coronavirus disease-2019 (COVID-19). *Indian J Pediatr.* 87(4):281–286.

10. Richman D.D., Whitley R.J., Hayden F.G. 2016. *Clinical Virology,* 4th ed. Washington, DC: ASM Press.

11. Camilla R., Schunk M., Sothmann P., et al. 2020. Transmission of 2019-nCoV infection from an asymptomatic contact in Germany. *N Engl J Med.* 382(10):970–971.

12. Zou L., Ruan F., Huang M., et al. 2020. SARS-CoV-2 viral load in upper respiratory specimens of infected patients. *N Engl J Med.* 12:1177–1179.

13. Kampf G., Todt D., Pfaender S., et al. 2020. Persistence of coronaviruses on inanimate surfaces and its inactivation with biocidal agents. *J Hosp Infect.* 104(3):246–251.

14. Huijun C., Guo J., Wang C., et al. 2020. Clinical characteristics and intrauterine vertical transmission potential of COVID-19 infection in nine pregnant women: a retrospective review of medical records. *Lancet* 395(10226):809–815.

15. Chen N., Zhou M., Dong X., et al. 2020. Epidemiological and clinical characteristics of 99 cases of 2019 novel coronavirus pneumonia in Wuhan, China: a descriptive study. *Lancet* 395:507–513.

16. Shi Y., Wang Y., Shao C., et al. 2020. COVID-19 infection: the perspectives on immune responses. *Cell Death Differ.* 27(5):1451–1454.

17. Deem M.W. 2005.Complexity in the immune system. *Comput Chem Eng.* 29(3):437–446.

18. Perelson A.S., Weisbuch G. 1997. Immunology for physicists. *Rev Mod Phys.* 69(4): 1219.

19. Simon H.B. 1984.The immunology of exercise: a brief review. *JAMA* 252(19):2735–2738.

20. Mainardi T., Kapoor S., Bielory L. 2009. Complementary and alternative medicine: herbs, phytochemicals and vitamins and their immunologic effects. *J Allergy Clin Immunol.* 123(2) 283–294.

21. Devasagayam T., Sainis K. 2002. Immune system and antioxidants, especially those derived from Indian medicinal plants. *Indian J Exp Biol.* 40:639–655.

22. Richart S.M. 2018. Synergic effect of curcumin and its structural analogue *(Monoacetylcurcumin)* on anti-influenza virus infection. *J Food Drug Anal.* 26(3):1015–1023.

23. Jagetia G.C., Aggarwal B.B. 2007. "Spicing up" of the immune system by curcumin. *J Clin Immunol.* 27(1):19–35.

24. Hemilä H. 2017. Vitamin C and infections. *Nutrients* 9(4):339.

25. Cannell J. 2006. Epidemic influenza and vitamin D. *Epidemiol Infect.* 134(6):1129–1140.

26. Shankar A.H., Prasad A.S. 1998. Zinc and immune function: the biological basis of altered resistance to infection. *Am J Clin Nutr.* 68(2):447S–463S.

27. Kempinska-Podhorodecka A. 2017.Decreased expression of vitamin D receptor affects an immune response in primary biliary cholangitis via the VDR-miRNA155-SOCS1 pathway. *Int J Mol Sci.* 18(2):289.
28. Administration, T.G. 2020. No evidence to support intravenous high-dose vitamin C in the management of COVID-19. https://www.tga.gov.au/alert/no-evidence-support-intravenous-high-dose-vitamin-c-management-covid-19.
29. Grant W.B. H. Lahore, S.L. McDonnell, C.A. Baggerly, C.B. French, J.L. Aliano, and H.P. Bhattoa. 2020. Evidence that vitamin D supplementation could reduce risk of influenza and COVID-19 infections and deaths. *Nutrients* 12: 988.
30. Nilashi M., Samad S., and Akbari E. 2020. Can complementary and alternative medicines be beneficial in the treatment of COVID-19 through improving immune system function?. *J Infect Public Health* 13(6):893–896.
31. Bloom, D.E., Cadarette D. 2019. Infectious disease threats in the twenty-first century: strengthening the global response. *Front Immunol.* 10:549.
32. Gray D.M., Joseph J.J., Olayiwola J.N. 2020. Strategies for digital care of vulnerable patients in a COVID-19 world – keeping in touch. *JAMA Health Forum* 1(6):e200734.
33. Hilbert M. 2011. The end justifies the definition: the manifold outlooks on the digital divide and their practical usefulness for policy-making. *Telecomm Policy* 35(8):715–736.
34. Zemencuk J.K., Hayward R.A., Skarupski K.A., et al. 1999. Patients' desires and expectations for medical care: a challenge to improving patient satisfaction. *Am J Med Qual.* 14(1):21–27.
35. Gordon H.S., Solanki P., Bokhour B.G., et al. 2020. "I'm not feeling like I'm part of the conversation" patients' perspectives on communicating in clinical video telehealth visits. *J Gen Intern Med.* 35(6):1751–1758.
36. Bauerly B.C., McCord R.F., Hulkower R., et al. 2019. Broadband access as a public health issue: the role of law in expanding broadband access and connecting underserved communities for better health outcomes. *J Law Med Ethics* 47(2 suppl):39–42.
37. Koh H.K., Gracia J.N., Alvarez M.E. 2014. Culturally and linguistically appropriate services – advancing health with CLAS. *N Engl J Med.* 371(3):198–201.
38. Norman C.D., Skinner H.A. 2006. eHealth literacy: essential skills for consumer health in a networked world. *J Med Internet Res.* 8(2):e9.
39. Lohr A.M., Ingram M., Nuñez A.V., et al. 2018. Community-clinical linkages with community health workers in the United States: a scoping review. *Health Promot Pract.* 19(3):349–360.
40. Moran M.E. 2007. Rossum's universal robots: not the machines. *J Endourol.* 21:1399–1402.
41. Neme R.M., Schraibman V., Okazaki S., et al. 2013. Deep infiltrating colorectal endometriosis treated with robotic-assisted rectosigmoidectomy. *JSLS* 17:227–234.
42. Chung Y., Zhu X., Gu W., et al. 2006. Microscale integrated sperm sorter. *Methods Mol Biol.* 321:227–244.
43. Perry T.S. 2013. Spectrum. *IEEE* 50:23.
44. Takanobu H., Okino A., Takanishi A., et al. 2006. *Dental Patient Robot.* Kolkata: Academic Publishers, pp. 1273–1278.
45. Kershner R.M. 2006. Could a robot soon replace your doctor? Seeing for life – everything you need to know for healthy eyes and clear vision. *Ocular Surgery News*, pp. 1–4.
46. Caballero-Morales S.O., Enríquez G.B., Romero F.T. 2013. Speech-based human and service robot interaction: an application for Mexican dysarthric people. *Int J Adv Robot Syst.* 10:1–14.
47. Bush B., Nifong L.W., Chitwood W.R. Jr. 2013. Robotics in cardiac surgery: past, present, and future. *Rambam Maimonides Med J.* 4:e0017.

48. O'Shaughnessy P.E. 2001. Introduction to forensic science. *Dent Clin North Am.* 45:217–227.
49. Thali M.J., Jackowski C., Oesterhelweg L., et al. 2007. Virtopsy – the Swiss virtual autopsy approach. *Leg Med (Tokyo).* 9:100–104.
50. Bolliger S.A., Thali M.J., Ross S., et al. 2008. Virtual autopsy using imaging: Bridging radiologic and forensic sciences. A review of the virtopsy and similar projects. *Eur Radiol.* 18:273–282.
51. Ebert L.C., Ptacek W., Naether S., et al. 2010. Virtobot – a multi-functional robotic system for 3D surface scanning and automatic post mortem biopsy. *Int J Med Robot.* 6:18–27.
52. Basheti I.A., Elayeh E.R., Al Natour D.B., et al. 2017. Opinions of pharmacists and herbalists on herbal medicine use and receiving herbal medicine education. *Jordan Trop J Pharm Res.* 16(3): 689–696.
53. Bhat B.B., Udupa N., Ligade V.S., et al. 2019, Assessment of knowledge and attitude of patients on herbal medicine use in Udupi region, Karnataka, India. *Trop J Pharm Res.* 18(1):117–121.
54. Kyegombe, W., Mutesi, R.I., Bakulumpagi, D., et al. 2016. Use of herbal medicines among pregnant women attending antenatal clinic at Kiryandogo General Hospital, Uganda. *East Afr Med J.* 93(10):536–541.
55. Mwangi, J.N., Mungai, N.N., ThoiThi, G.N., et al. (n.d.). Traditional herbal medicine in National Healthcare in Kenya. *East Central Afr J Pharm Sci.* 8(2):22–26.
56. Tshibangu, K.C., Worku, Z.B., De Jongh, M.A., et al. 2004. Assessment of effectiveness of traditional herbal medicine in managing HIV/AIDs patients in South Africa. *East Afr Med J.* 81(10):499–504.
57. Sanderoff, B.T. Winter 2000–2001. Herbal medicine: use with caution and respect. *J Am Soc Aging.* 24(4):69–74.
58. Vickers, A. and Zollman. C. 1999. ABC of complementary medicine: herbal medicine. *BMJ* 319(7216):1050–1053.
59. Martin, A.J. and Marsh, H.W. 2003. Fear of failure: Friend or foe? *Aust. Psychol.* 38:31–38.

4 ASBGo: A Smart Walker for Ataxic Gait and Posture Assessment, Monitoring, and Rehabilitation

*João M. Lopes, João André, António Pereira,
Manuel Palermo, and Nuno Ribeiro*
University of Minho

João Cerqueira
Clinical Academic Center (2CA-Braga),
Hospital of Braga, Braga, Portugal

Cristina P. Santos
University of Minho

CONTENTS

INTRODUCTION

Disability is inherent to the human condition. According to the World Health Organization (WHO), more than one billion people suffer from a form of disability, arising to nearly 15% of the world's population, and the number is still growing (World Health Organization 2011a). Dysfunctional gait, for instance, is the most common disability among European countries, where it is estimated that more than 5 million people are dependent on a wheelchair (Mikolajczyk et al. 2018). This is because of the aging population, but also because of the increased incidence of neurological disorders worldwide (Meng et al. 2015).

Cerebellar ataxia is a neurological condition that strongly affects the patient's mobility, affecting motor coordination, postural control, and spatiotemporal awareness (Ilg and Timmann 2013; Ilg et al. 2007; Buckley, Mazzà, and McNeill 2018). It results in damage to the cerebellum or its afferent pathways (Ilg and Timmann 2013) due to inherited or acquired causes (Buckley, Mazzà, and McNeill 2018), such as stroke. Besides other functionalities, the cerebellum plays an important role in gait and postural control, by regulating the movement of the limbs and coordinating the muscles' activation (Ilg and Timmann 2013). Typical ataxic gait is characterized by an unstable and stumbling walk, mainly caused by the lack of multi-joint coordination (dysmetria) and the deficit in maintaining postural control (Ilg and Timmann 2013; Ilg et al. 2007), strongly restricting patients' mobility and increasing the risk of falls (Fonteyn et al. 2010). Consequently, their quality of life is highly jeopardized, affecting their daily life activities and their social and work well-being (Moreira et al. 2019). Besides, mobility restrictions cause social-economic consequences, namely the increasing of health and social costs with the high institutionalization and dependence on a third party (Moreira et al. 2019). Since there is neither a pharmacological nor a surgical solution that completely restores the neurological damages and reverses the motor disabilities of cerebellar ataxia patients (Moreira et al. 2019; Milne et al. 2017), rehabilitation is the keyword (Moreira et al. 2019).

Recent works have been studying the effects of rehabilitation in persons with some type of ataxia. Its effectiveness is still a paradigm to research and needs further investigation. An effective comprehension of the rehabilitation effects may enable the development of effective, time-efficient, and user-oriented therapies (Milne et al. 2017). Milne et al. (2017) showed that patients with ataxia demonstrated a significant improvement in, at least, one outcome. Magaña et al. (Tercero-Pérez et al. 2019) also studied the effects of physical rehabilitation in patients with spinocerebellar ataxia type 7. The authors found that moderated and intensive training allowed a significant improvement in the SARA (scale for the assessment and rating of ataxia) score when compared with the control group, with special emphasis on SARA sub-scores regarding gait and dysmetria (Tercero-Pérez et al. 2019).

Rehabilitation therapies involve high-skilled professionals of different areas and their effectiveness relies on the therapist's experience (Mikolajczyk et al. 2018). Furthermore, current rehabilitation scenarios entail a high burden of care to clinicians and the patient's assessment is based on subjective metrics instead of objective parameters (World Health Organization 2011b). Therefore, biomedical research is sought for creating complementary means of rehabilitation to (i) promote motor skills learning and training to patients; (ii) reduce the heavy burden of manual therapy to clinicians; (iii) provide repetitive and intensity-adapted rehabilitation scenarios; and (iv) reduce the palliative care and institutionalization costs (Mikolajczyk et al. 2018; Moreira et al. 2019). Walkers and canes were one of the solutions. Nearly 7 million persons use canes or walkers as mobility aids just in the United States of America (Bateni and Maki 2005). Conventional walkers, for instance, improve the patient's static and dynamic stability by offering a base of support (Bradley and Hernandez 2011; Neto et al. 2015). For cerebellar ataxic patients, this base of support is of utmost importance given their symptomatology of poor balance and multiarticular coordination. However, such assistive devices should be tailored to each patient. According to Bateni and Maki (2005), between 30% and 50% of users stop using their mobility aids. Many causes may explain this behavior, but inappropriate device prescription or self-prescribed assistive devices and inadequate user training may be the probable cause (Bateni and Maki 2005). Moreover, conventional walkers are associated with an increased risk of falls and may augment the user's walking energy expenditure (Neto et al. 2015). Therefore, there is a considerable need for advanced rehabilitation devices that not only provide patients with repetitive and effective therapies, but also provide them stability, confidence, and safety, and release clinicians from the burden of manual therapy. A solution is the multifunctional robotic walkers that combine safety and ergonomics to deliver proper assist-as-need assistance to their end-users. According to WHO, assistive technologies have shown promising results in providing independence and improving the patients' participation in their rehabilitation therapies (World Health Organization 2011b). The goal of these assistive technologies is to improve the patients' mobility by fostering a human–robot interaction and cooperation that empowers the user's recovery state (Bradley and Hernandez 2011).

This chapter presents the current paradigm of smart walkers as multifunctional assistive devices that intend to aid the elderly and/or motor-impaired persons. Their functionalities, benefits, and limitations will be further discussed, presenting the status. Furthermore, the ASBGo Smart Walker will be presented. A journey from the beginnings of this project to present will be performed, presenting the structural and functional modifications all over the years. Finally, the main conclusions and future insights will be discussed.

WALKERS AS AIDS OF LOCOMOTION

Walkers have assumed an important role as an aid of locomotion due to their simplicity, comfort, and potential to be used in rehabilitation scenarios (Neto et al. 2015; Martins et al. 2012). These devices avoid the early use of wheelchairs (potentially decreasing institutionalization and third-party dependence costs) by using the person's residual motor skills to augment their locomotion. These devices are often referred to as augmentative devices since they empower the end-user physical and cognitive capabilities (Neto et al. 2015; Martins et al. 2012). By providing a base of support, gait assistance, and postural control, walkers are one of the most used assistive devices worldwide. Besides residual motor improvements, investigations have shown that these devices can provide other physiological improvements, namely at the cardiorespiratory and skeletal levels (Bateni and Maki 2005; Neto et al. 2015; Martins et al. 2012).

Walkers can be divided into conventional and smart walkers depending on their mechanical structure and functionalities. Conventional walkers are intended to be only walking assistants (passive device), while smart walkers are intended to join the advantages of conventional walkers, overcome their limitations, and bring other relevant features, such as health monitoring, cognitive assistance, and human–robot interaction (active device) (Martins et al. 2012).

CONVENTIONAL WALKERS

There are three types of conventional walkers, depending on their mechanical structure: (i) the standard walker, (ii) the two-wheeled walker, and (iii) the four-wheeled walker, also named as rollator (Bradley and Hernandez 2011; Neto et al. 2015; Martins et al. 2012). The standard walker is the most known worldwide. It is a simple metallic structure with four contacts to the ground. From the three types of conventional walkers, it is considered the most stable since it provides a strong base of support (Bradley and Hernandez 2011). Nevertheless, it entails high coordination and control when lifting the device from the ground to perform the walking steps (Neto et al. 2015). This requires a higher effort on the upper limbs, which is not adequate for motor-impaired individuals, particularly for ataxic patients, leading to early fatigue (Neto et al. 2015). Since cerebellar ataxia strongly affects the ability of patients to maintain postural control, the standard walker is not the most clinically suited. Moreover, lifting the device from the ground may cause an additional risk of fall (Bateni and Maki 2005).

The two-wheeled walker is an evolution of the standard walker. Its mechanical structure is similar, but it was added two wheels at the front to provide a more dynamic comfort. With this mechanical difference regarding the standard walker, the patients do not need to lift the device from the ground to walk forward. This characteristic provides the user with a more natural gait pattern, with increased gait speed. By not lifting the device from the ground, it does not entail a higher effort when compared with the standard walker, but current evidence shows that this solution is less stable for motor-impaired patients (Bradley and Hernandez 2011; Neto et al. 2015).

At last, the four-wheeled walker, also named rollator, is more intended for those patients that do not need a wider base of support (Bradley and Hernandez 2011). Besides being more energetically efficient, this is not the most suitable solution for ataxic patients since it can roll forward without the patient's intention (Bradley and Hernandez 2011; Neto et al. 2015). Moreover, the braking system needs some dexterity, ability, and good reaction time that, for some patients with cognitive impairments, may result in an increased difficulty (Martins et al. 2012).

SMART WALKERS

Besides the advantages of conventional walkers, they present some limitations that lead to the open investigation of new resources and means of attaining the patients' effective assistance and rehabilitation by following a more user-centered approach that gathers safety and comfort. With this statement in mind, the biomedical investigation presented the smart walkers, an evolution of conventional walkers that gather the concepts of medical robotics, control, and automation to create fully assistive devices with numerous functionalities. These include (i) stability and physical support, (ii) decoding user's motion intention, (iii) navigation assistance, (iv) sensorial feedback and health monitoring, and (v) safety mechanisms (Martins et al. 2012). Table 4.1 presents some of the current smart walkers of literature, their sensors, modes of operation, and functionalities.

Stability and Physical Support

Physical support is an important functionality for motor-impaired patients. For ataxic patients, smart walkers must provide means of body weight support, providing users with static and dynamic stability (Mun et al. 2017). A study that gathered 100 stroke patients had shown that gait training associated with body-weight support improved the patients' walking speed, functional balance, and motor recovery (Barbeau and Visintin 2003). By providing body-weight support, the patients will have increased stability by reducing the gravitational forces that act on the body, improving the postural sway (Mun et al. 2017). Most robotic walkers of literature (see Table 4.1) comprise handles as the conventional walkers do, but i-Walker (Annicchiarico et al. 2008; Cortés et al. 2008), JARoW (Lee, Ohnuma, and Chong 2010; Lee et al. 2011), Simbiosis (Frizera-Neto et al. 2011), and UFES (Neto et al. 2015; Jiménez et al. 2019) walkers provide forearms supports on their mechanical structure on which patients can rely.

User's Motion Intention Decoding

In robotics-based rehabilitation, human–robot cooperation and interaction are important to attain effective rehabilitation (Beckerle et al. 2017). Decoding the user's motion intention is one type of human–robot interaction. Most of the robotic walkers of literature provide a human–machine interface to control the device. The user's intention is decoded mainly with force sensors, either placed on the handles or placed on the forearms support. With this physical/direct interaction, the user's intention is converted into guidance commands of walking forward, turning left, or turning right. This could be interpreted as the walker manual guidance in which the user is

TABLE 4.1
Smart Walkers Presented in the Literature and Their Respective Target Population, Sensors, Mode(s) of Operation and Functionalities

Study	Target Population	Sensors	Modes of Operation	Functionalities
PAMM (Spenko, Yu, and Dubowsky 2006)	Elderly	Sonar, camera, force sensor	User-control, path following	Obstacle avoidance, localization, and health monitoring
GUIDO (Lacey and Rodriguez-Losada 2008; Rentschler et al. 2008)	Visually impaired	Laser, sonar, force sensor	User-control, autonomous mode	Voice command, obstacle avoidance, localization, navigation, decode user's intention
i-Walker (Annicchiarico et al. 2008; Cortés et al. 2008)	Elderly and motor-impaired	Force sensor, inclinometer	User-control, cooperative mode, adaptive mode	Decode user's intention, user's fall-aware, path planning, navigation, safety mechanism
JARoW (Lee, Ohnuma, and Chong 2010; Lee et al. 2011)	Elderly	Infrared sensor, laser	User-control	Gait detection, obstacle detection
Simbiosis (Frizera-Neto et al. 2011)	Elderly and motor-impaired	Force sensor, sonar	User-control	Physical support, decode user's intention, gait monitoring
CAIROW (Chang et al. 2012)	Parkinson's patients	Laser, camera, force sensor	User-control, autonomous mode	Decode user's intention, obstacle detection, graphical user interface, localization, path planning, and navigation

(Continued)

TABLE 4.1 (CONTINUED)

Smart Walkers Presented in the Literature and Their Respective Target Population, Sensors, Mode(s) of Operation and Functionalities

Study	Target Population	Sensors	Modes of Operation	Functionalities
UFES (Neto et al. 2015; Jiménez et al. 2019)	Elderly and motor-impaired	IMU[a], laser, force sensor	User-control	Physical support, decode user's intention, visual feedback for path following, obstacle detection, gait monitoring
N/A (Ye et al. 2012; Huang et al. 2015)	Elderly	Force sensor, IMU[a]	User-control	Gait recognition, fall detection, safety mechanisms
MOBOT (Efthimiou et al. 2016)	Elderly	Force sensor, laser, cameras, microphone	User-control and autonomous	Sit-to-stand, stand-to-sit assistance, voice command, gesture recognition, fall detection, navigation, obstacle avoidance, physiological monitoring
ISR-AIWALKER (Paulo, Peixoto, and Nunes 2017)	Motor-impaired	Infrared and RGB-D cameras	User-control, navigation assistance	Decode user's intention, gait monitoring and analysis, gait classification, navigation assistance
AGoRA (Sierra et al. 2018, 2019)	Elderly and motor-impaired	Laser, sonar, force sensor, camera	User-control, supervised and autonomous	Decode user's intention, detect user's presence and support, localization, path planning, and navigation, obstacle detection, gait monitoring
FriWalk (Ferrari et al. 2020)	Elderly	Camera	User-control and robot-control	Navigation assistance with shared control

[a] *Inertial measurement unit.*

under control of the device. For instance, PAAM (Spenko, Yu, and Dubowsky 2006), GUIDO (Lacey and Rodriguez-Losada 2008; Rentschler et al. 2008), i-Walker (Annicchiarico et al. 2008; Cortés et al. 2008), CAIROW (Chang et al. 2012), and the walker proposed in Ye et al. (2012) and Huang et al. (2015), comprise 3D force sensors on the handlebars to directly measure the force/torque the user is applying. Other works, namely Simbiosis (Frizera-Neto et al. 2011) and UFES (Neto et al. 2015; Jiménez et al. 2019) walkers, take advantage of having body-weight support and coupled force sensors at the forearms support. The force that is applied to the forearms support is divided into the tree-axis to assess the user's intention and guide the walker accordingly. A recent work, AGoRA walker (Sierra et al. 2018, 2019), also employs a human–robot interaction using force sensors, but these are not directly applied on the handlebars. Instead, the force sensors are coupled to the mechanical structure of the walker. The forces that users apply on the force sensors are usually interpreted by an admittance controller. However, some works of literature consider that the use of force sensors is not the most reliable solution in the long term since they present hysteresis and may degrade with time (Paulo, Peixoto, and Nunes 2017).

Therefore, some different approaches relying on cameras, infrared sensors, and lasers have been presented. For instance, JARoW contains two infrared sensors on its mechanical structure that points toward the end-user shin (Lee, Ohnuma, and Chong 2010; Lee et al. 2011). The user's motion intention is decoded indirectly by assessing the shin's location in space. Another interesting work is that presented in Paulo, Peixoto, and Nunes (2017), ISR-AIWALKER, that uses a Leap Motion device below the handlebars to detect their displacement and, based on a fuzzy-logic controller, the guidance commands are generated. Other walkers, namely PAAM (Spenko, Yu, and Dubowsky 2006), GUIDO (Lacey and Rodriguez-Losada 2008; Rentschler et al. 2008), and MOBOT (Efthimiou et al. 2016) present voice commands strategies, which are useful for visually impaired patients. However, the effectiveness of this solution is limited by the environmental context, which could potentiate noise that makes speech recognition difficult (Moreira et al. 2019).

Navigation Assistance

Navigation assistance is an important feature that walkers for rehabilitation can provide, by helping their end-users with their navigation and localization. Some neurological disorders can also affect the memory of patients and their spatio-temporal awareness. Therefore, this functionality is particularly interesting for this kind of patients since, in this way, they can truly focus on their rehabilitation therapy without having the concern of guiding the system elsewhere (Moreira et al. 2019). As such, many robotic walkers of literature are equipped with a considerable number of sensors, namely ultrasonic sensors, lasers, and cameras, giving walkers the ability to localize, map, and drive autonomously. Along with this functionality, walkers are also capable of detecting obstacles and, in some cases, preventing a collision by giving an alternative path or making an emergency stop. PAMM walker, for instance, contains an array of ultrasonic sensors and one camera. The camera is facing upwards since signposts are on the ceiling for localization. The device is able to communicate with a central computer that facilitates the environment map and alerts for any permanent obstacles (Spenko, Yu, and Dubowsky 2006). GUIDO walker is another walker that employs this functionality by using ultrasonic sensors and a laser range finder. The walker can build the environment map in real time through a simultaneous localization and mapping (SLAM) algorithm, using the information gathered with the laser placed on the front of the walker (Lacey and Rodriguez-Losada 2008; Rentschler et al. 2008). Other walkers, such as CAIROW, MOBOT, and AGoRA walkers, also provide a similar strategy.

Recently, some works of literature have adopted a shared control between walker and user, consisting of another type of human–robot interaction and cooperation (Ye et al. 2018). The main goal is to create harmony between humans and machines in which the machine aids the user only when needed – an assist-as-needed strategy. For instance, the PAMM walker (Spenko, Yu, and Dubowsky 2006) employs an adaptive shared control in which the walker's central control unit assesses the user's performance and decides if the user is guiding the system safely or if the user is correctly guiding the walker throughout the planned path. Based on the user's performance, the adaptation law adapts the gains on the user's contribution and the walker assistance, which is fed into an admittance controller responsible for generating the guidance commands (Spenko, Yu, and Dubowsky 2006). GUIDO, COOL Aide (Huang et al. 2005), and AGoRA walkers also provide a shared control strategy. A different approach was presented for the ISR-AIWALKER in which the walker evaluates the local environment using an RGB-D camera. With this information, the walker perceives if the user's intention is considered safe navigation or not. If not, the shared control provides an adequate response toward a safe route (Paulo, Peixoto, and Nunes 2017; Paulo 2017).

Sensorial Feedback and Health Monitoring

Another relevant functionality for patient rehabilitation that smart walkers should provide is sensorial feedback and health monitoring (Paulo, Peixoto, and Nunes 2017). As previously mentioned, patients are currently assessed using subjective metrics, such as the SARA (Schmitz-Hübsch et al. 2006) and the Berg balance scale (Berg et al. 1992). These were proved to be reliable, but there is a lack of objective metrics assessment and their relationship with the clinical scales. As a rehabilitation device, smart walkers should be used as therapy tools, providing a full gait and posture analysis. With this information, the clinicians may monitor their users over time and prescribe adequate functional rehabilitation therapies accordingly (Moreira et al. 2019).

Some walkers of literature provide this functionality. For instance, the Simbiosis walker makes use of ultrasonic sensors to measure the user's feet evolution by assessing the feet's distance to the walker. Moreover, using the force sensors on the forearms supports, the authors also estimate gait cadence (Frizera-Neto et al. 2011). Gait cadence is also estimated by the UFES walker using a laser range finder that measures the feet's evolution when walking with the assistive walker (Neto et al. 2015;

Jiménez et al. 2019; Cifuentes et al. 2016). A similar approach was employed on the JARoW walker using infrared sensors (Lee, Ohnuma, and Chong 2010; Lee et al. 2011). On the author side, a wearable solution is proposed comprising inertial measurement units to estimate posture in real time (Ye et al. 2012; Huang et al. 2015). The posture is analyzed by calculating the center-of-gravity using a HAT (head-arms-torso) configuration (Ye et al. 2012; Huang et al. 2015). At last, the ISR-AIWALKER presents a more detailed algorithm for gait analysis by using a leap motion controller and an RGB-D camera. The authors present an algorithm capable of performing the gait cycle segmentation by detecting the heel-strike event. Moreover, the walker also provides hip and knee joint angles (Paulo, Peixoto, and Nunes 2017). Another approach using the camera's information was presented by Lim et al. (2016), whose information is used to calculate spatiotemporal parameters such as the stride length, step length, and step velocity. Nevertheless, this topic still needs further investigation due to the high variability of gait and postural sway induced by motor disabilities.

Gait and posture information can be used to give biofeedback to patients. Although there is a lack of studies reporting significant improvements in rehabilitation using biofeedback, recent evidence classifies its use as promising (Giggins, Persson, and Caulfield 2013; Stanton et al. 2017; van Gelder et al. 2018). A search on the literature reports a lack of biofeedback use along with robotic walkers. Along with the ASBGo Smart Walker, the walker proposed by Lim et al. (2016) provides visual cues projected on the floor and rhythmic sounds to encourage the users to move forward. The authors reported an improvement of 30% in stride length by using biofeedback. Further investigation on this topic should be carried out since it is considered of utmost importance to the patients' rehabilitation.

Safety Mechanisms

Safety mechanisms are important when dealing with persons with motor disabilities. Their gait is typically irregular increasing the number of falls and, consequently, fall-related morbidities. Most of the smart walkers in literature, and those on Table 4.1, provide embedded safety mechanisms.

The most common observed in the literature is obstacle detection and avoidance. By taking advantage of their embedded sensors, mostly sonars, and laser range finders, smart walkers can map their surrounding environment, detecting permanent and punctual obstacles that may compromise the patients' safety. A collision with an obstacle may provide instability to the patient, causing their fall. For instance, the PAAM (Spenko, Yu, and Dubowsky 2006), GUIDO (Lacey and Rodriguez-Losada 2008; Rentschler et al. 2008), JARoW (Lee, Ohnuma, and Chong 2010; Lee et al. 2011), CAIROW (Chang et al. 2012), UFES (Neto et al. 2015; Jiménez et al. 2019), MOBOT (Efthimiou et al. 2016), and AGoRA (Sierra et al. 2018, 2019) walkers present this functionality. Some of these walkers also use shared control as a safety mechanism, prioritizing the users' control over the smart walker until a dangerous situation is detected. Examples are PAAM (Spenko, Yu, and Dubowsky 2006) and FriWalk (Ferrari et al. 2020) walkers.

Another common safety mechanism of smart walkers is to not allow patients to walk backward. The wheels are locked and do not allow such movement to prevent users from falling backward. JARoW is one example that contemplates this safety mechanism (Lee, Ohnuma, and Chong 2010; Lee et al. 2011).

Recently, some walkers of literature are providing safety mechanisms to prevent users from falling by immediately stopping the walker whenever a near-fall is detected. For instance, the walker proposed by Taghvaei, Hirata, and Kosuge (2010) and Taghvaei and Kosuge (2018) presents vision-based algorithms for tracking the upper body and classifies the fall. Another approach involving force-sensing resistors and laser range finders was presented by Xu, Huang, and Cheng (2018) along with a support vector machine to detect whenever a fall may occur. On the other side, Huang et al. used a different approach (Ye et al. 2012; Huang et al. 2015). Wearable and non-wearable sensors were used to detect possible falls, while in other works, only non-wearable sensors were used. A tri-axial accelerometer, a tri-axial magnetometer, and a tri-axial gyroscope were positioned on the waist, two thighs, and two shanks to calculate the acceleration and the angular velocity. The fuzzy threshold was the approach implemented to detect the fall. When the fall is detected, the walker brakes.

In the following section, the ASBGo Smart Walker will be presented. Its architecture, design, functionalities, and clinical evidence will be presented and discussed. Future research insights will also be presented.

ASBGO: SYSTEM OVERVIEW, ARCHITECTURE, FUNCTIONALITIES, AND FUTURE PERSPECTIVES

Many smart walkers have been presented in the literature to satisfy the limitations of conventional walkers. However, further investigation is needed on this topic to obtain an effective device based on (i) personalization, aiming the best rehabilitation practices by understanding and customizing the therapy to the users' needs and considering their residual capabilities, and (ii) human–robot interaction that maximizes the cooperation between patient and machine, increasing their motivation and participation on the rehabilitation therapy.

This section presents the ASBGo Smart Walker. The system overview will be presented, focusing on the system's mechanical structure and architecture, and its main functionalities.

FROM PROTOTYPE I TO ASBGO

When designing a smart walker intended for the rehabilitation of persons with motor disabilities, a list of goals should be addressed to specify all the requirements needed. The main goal is to guarantee the safety of the end-user, creating a robust and reliable walker. The second goal is to achieve a multifunctional device that is fully adjusted to the users' needs and requirements and able to incorporate several key technologies that are relevant to attain current challenges of the state-of-the-art, such as continuous gait and posture assessment, assist-as-needed strategies that foster a compliant and interactive human–robot cooperation, and biofeedback to improve and enhance residual motor skills. The ASBGo Smart Walker rises from these challenges, comprising numerous functionalities to provide effective and time-efficient rehabilitation.

ASBGo is a smart, personalized, and user-oriented four-wheeled motorized walker that provides assistance and rehabilitation to ataxic patients. It contains numerous embedded sensors that transform it into an ambulatory device for motor assessment and rehabilitation. The project counts with four prototypes, as illustrated in Figure 4.1. They evolved by following a user-centered approach considering innumerous brainstorms with the team's engineers and clinicians to develop the most ergonomic and personalized device, maximizing its usability.

The first prototype (Prototype I) was considered a proof-of-concept (Martins, Santos, and Frizera 2012). It was based on a heavy rudimental structure with little evolved electronics, presenting delay and hysteresis on its behavior. The second prototype (Prototype II) presented an improvement in the mechanical structure and was the first to be tested in a real environment along with ataxic patients (Martins et al. 2014). It was lighter, easy to use, easy to transport and store, but it was limited in personalization and adjustments to the end-user. The third prototype (ASBGo III) was more ergonomic and stable. Two horizontal handlebars were introduced to assist patients in standing and stand-to-sit movements and a table of wood was introduced to support the users' weight. The structure also allowed for mechanical adjustments on height, fostering a more user-centered design; however, the system had some limitations given the type of materials that were chosen (aluminum) (Alves et al. 2016). The fourth and current prototype (ASBGo++, ASBGo*) had significant improvements in mechanics and electronics. A renewed mechanical structure was manufactured based on more resistant materials (stainless steel) (Alves et al. 2016). Despite being more cumbersome, this structure was revealed to be more stable and stronger. It was designed to fully attain the end-user requirements, raising considerably the level of customization and acceptance of the final product. The mechanical system for height adjustment was replaced by two electric lifting systems (see Figure 4.2D), capable of withstanding a maximum admissible load of 800 N ($\approx$ 81.6 kgf), allowing a full user-oriented device that provides dynamic stability while maintaining a correct posture. Furthermore, the wood platform (see Figure 4.2M) was redesigned to provide more space and ergonomics to the end-user forearms. Lastly, a harness (see Figure 4.2N) was also introduced to provide more safety and confidence to the end-user while walking with the assistive device.

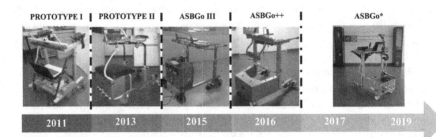

FIGURE 4.1 Chronological evolution of the ASBGo Smart Walker.

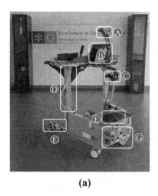 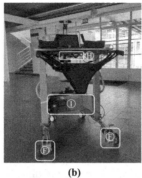 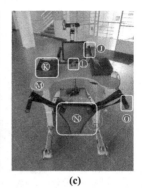

(a) (b) (c)

FIGURE 4.2 ASBGo's views: (a) front, (b) rear, and (c) top. The fifth prototype will have minor modifications to the mechanical structure. It will pass to a three-wheel configuration to provide more maneuverability while maintaining the patient's stability. The prototype includes (A) RGB-D camera for posture analysis, (B) touch screen, (C) RGB-D camera for gait analysis, (D) an electric lifting system, (E) main CCU, (F) DC motors, (G) laser and sonar sensors, (H) infrared sensor, (I) electronics box compartment, (J) specially designed handlebar, (K) force sensors on the forearms support, (L) emergency button, (M) ergonomic wood table for body-weight support, (N) harness, and (O) horizontal handles for standing and stand-to-sit assistance.

System Overview

Figure 4.2 presents the ASBGo current prototype, considering the front, rear, and top view. The smart walker is composed of two motorized rear wheels (24 V DC motor with a nominal speed of 40 rpm and a nominal torque of 5 Nm, see Figure 4.2F) coupled with an encoder. The front wheels are passive (caster-wheels) and move according to the desired direction. Each motor is controlled independently using a dedicated architecture, allowing it to move forward, turn left, and turn right. Additionally, they can be decoupled from the wheels if needed, becoming a fully passive device, to facilitate transportation within the clinical facilities. The device is controlled using a user-friendly and ergonomic handlebar (Figure 4.2J) and fed with two 12V rechargeable batteries. The handlebar, consisting of a spring-based system with embedded potentiometers, was specially designed to fulfill the patients' morbidities, and it is responsible to directly decode the users' motion intention (Alves et al. 2016).

The smart walker is composed of numerous embedded sensors, namely RGB-D cameras (Figure 4.2A and C), ultrasonic sensors (Figure 4.2G), a laser range finder sensor (Figure 4.2G), and an infrared sensor (Figure 4.2H), that will allow the user's continuous monitorization and the implementation of safety strategies. Additionally, the smart walker contains an external IMU to estimate the center-of-mass (COM) and perform a biomechanical analysis.

ASBGo also includes a dedicated touch screen (Figure 4.2B) that runs a user-friendly graphical user interface (GUI), interacting with both the patient and clinician by allowing the therapy settings (e.g., insert a patient, create a session, activate/deactivate sensors, generate reports, select gait speed, select curvature, among others)

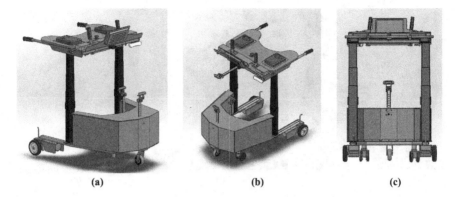

(a) (b) (c)

FIGURE 4.3 Fifth prototype of ASBGo: (a) right side, (b) left side, and (c) rear side. The mechanical structure will suffer minor modifications to allow the user to use the device with three and four wheels.

and providing other functionalities, such as the multitasking games and biofeedback activation.

A fifth prototype is currently under development, and it will provide improvements on the device's usability and functionality. The mechanical structure will have minor modifications but will allow the device's functionality within three or four wheels, as illustrated in Figure 4.3. The modification for three wheels will provide higher maneuverability while maintaining the patient's stability. Additionally, the handlebar will also be modified to provide higher flexibility and maneuverability for ataxic patients. The joystick will be bidirectional, allowing both linear and rotational movements.

System Architecture

The software architecture follows a modular and hierarchical architecture divided into high- and low-level controls. It was designed to be easily interpreted and changed if necessary when adding new functionalities and operating modes. This hierarchical approach is a very common architecture and transversal to other types of assistive devices, such as orthoses and prostheses (Tucker et al. 2015). Figure 4.4 illustrates ASBGo's renewed architecture.

The low-level control is considered the execution layer (Tucker et al. 2015). It runs a real-time operating system (RTOS) on an STM32F4 Discovery. Currently, this dedicated board is used to operate and read the smart walker low-level sensors and for controlling the device in terms of linear and angular speed, activating/deactivating the motors considering the response of a PID controller. This controller is responsible to generate an adequate response considering the deviation between the measured and the reference speed. The low-level sensors include the ultrasonic sensors (Figure 4.2G), the linear and angular potentiometers embedded on the handlebar (Figure 4.2J), the infrared sensor (Figure 4.2H), the encoders of each rear wheel (Figure 4.2F), the load cell (Figure 4.2K), and the emergency button (Figure 4.2L).

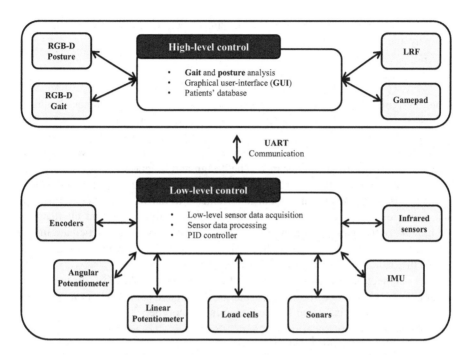

FIGURE 4.4 ASBGo renewed and modular architecture design. It is divided into high- and low-level controls, where the high-level control is responsible for the device's central control and the low-level control is responsible for data acquisition, processing, and the PID controller.

Each sensor is responsible for one or more functionalities of ASBGo that will be detailed in the next section.

The ultrasonic sensors are used for safety mechanisms by detecting punctual obstacles that are near the device and expose the user to risks. The linear and angular potentiometers are used to detect the user's motion intention and translate this intention into a measurable variable. The infrared sensor is located immediately above the wood platform and points directly to the user. It is used to assess the user's distance relative to the device. The encoders of each wheel are used to estimate the device's speed so that it is possible to control the device by comparing the measured speed with the reference speed selected on the GUI. The load cells are located in the elbow pads to measure the interaction and amount of weight the user is applying on the device. At last, the emergency button is used as a safety mechanism that cuts the power supply of both DC motors, allowing an emergency stop.

The high-level control, on the other side, is intended to establish the bridge between humans and machines. It runs in an Intel NUC computer over a ROS (robot operating system) layer, and it is considered the device's central control unit. It has three sensors connected directly to this level, namely two RGB-D cameras and one laser range finder. With the information gathered with the two RGB-D cameras, the high-level control is responsible for running computer vision-based algorithms for gait and posture assessment and monitorization. Moreover, it is responsible for receiving and interpreting the control commands when the device is controlled both remotely and autonomously.

FUNCTIONALITIES

When designing a smart walker, some challenges and key technologies should be addressed. Through a state-of-the-art analysis, personalization is of utmost importance and the most difficult challenge to overcome. Smart walkers should be able to fulfill the end-user requirements considering his/her disability level, fostering effective and time-efficient assistance. The design and functionalities should be outlined by following a human-centered design, involving since early the end-user in the design process, raising individual requirements to deliver a customized therapy that enhances the patients' residual motor skills. Another important challenge is the human–robot interaction that encourages the user to actively participate in his/her therapy. This can be accomplished with bio-inspired assistive technologies that ensure the patient's contribution to the rehabilitation.

This sub-section presents the current functionalities of ASBGo, discussing its advantages and limitations beyond the state-of-the-art and presenting future perspectives that are being considered for the upcoming prototype.

Users' Motion Intention Decoding

Decoding the users' motion intention is important to provide users the ability to guide the smart walker whenever they want to go, fostering human–robot cooperation intuitively. One of the main limitations of the state-of-the-art for conventional walkers is the maneuverability of such devices when dealing with persons with motor impairments. Smart walkers improve this maneuverability by using embedded sensors, such as force sensors on the handlebars, directly measuring the users' motion intention, and cameras and infrared sensors, without offering a high cognitive load and effort.

Given the high variability of ataxic gait, vision-based techniques may not be suited to decode the user's motion intentions, especially in the early beginnings of the rehabilitation therapy, in which patients present a stumbled and very unstable walk. Therefore, a specially designed handlebar was developed for the ASBGo Smart Walker. This handlebar contains two embedded sensors: (i) a linear potentiometer (0–10 kΩ) to detect directional changes in speed and (ii) a rotary potentiometer (0–470 kΩ) to detect forward changes in speed. According to the user's intention to move forward or turning right or left, the smart walker interprets this intention using fuzzy logic to classify the signals and control the motors' speed.

Results and Discussion

Figure 4.5 illustrates an example of the linear and rotary potentiometers when facing three activities: (i) walking forward (A), (ii) walking forward while turning left (B), and (iii) walking forward and turning right (C). Figure 4.5 also illustrates (a) the percentage of both rotary potentiometer (dashed line) and linear potentiometer (continuous line) and (b) the percentage of motors' velocity for both left (dashed line) and right (continuous line) motors.

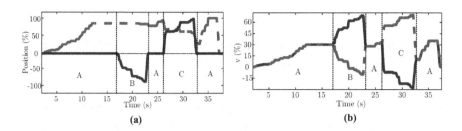

FIGURE 4.5 (a) Percentage of rotary potentiometer movement (dashed line) and the percentage of linear potentiometer movement (continuous line). (b) Percentage of the left motor (dashed line) and right motor (continuous line) velocity.

Analyzing Figure 4.5, the percentage of rotary position assumes a higher and positive value during activity A, indicating that the user wants to move forward. On the other side, the linear potentiometer assumes the value 0%, indicating that the users do not intend to change the smart walker's direction (turning right or turning left). This motion intention is traduced to a walking command, augmenting the motors' speed, as depicted in Figure 4.5b. In both activities B and C, the linear potentiometer presents a relative displacement regarding its original value, indicating the intention of changing the movement's direction. This displacement generates a control command that is sent to the low-level control and changes the motors' speed, allowing the device to turn.

This specially designed handlebar revealed promising, fostering human–robot cooperation and interaction ergonomically and intuitively. Nevertheless, the manual operation mode should only be used in patients with enough cognitive and visual capabilities, and upper-limb coordination. If these requirements are not fulfilled, ASBGo also provides a navigation assistance mode.

Navigation Assistance

Considering the patients' level of disability, ASBGo provides three modes of operation, as presented in Table 4.2: (i) manual guidance, which was discussed above, (ii) the autonomous mode, and (iii) the remote control. The navigation assistance functionality comprises the autonomous and remote-control modes.

The autonomous mode can be used when patients exhibit visual and cognitive limitations that make it impossible to drive the smart walker safely. With this operation mode, the clinician sets different types of rehabilitation scenarios and the walker drives itself without needing constant supervision. A local navigation module based on a non-linear dynamical system approach (DSA) with obstacle avoidance was implemented using the embedded ultrasonic sensors (Silva, Santos, and Sequeira 2013; Faria et al. 2014). The results demonstrated that the sonar configuration had successfully detected both dynamic and permanent obstacles. Real experiments in a laboratory context can be found in Martins, Faria, et al. (2015). Currently, the team improved the autonomous mode using the embedded laser range finder (Moreira et al. 2019).

The remote control is another ASBGo functionality. This mode of operation was designed to allow the clinician to control the device when needed, guiding the

TABLE 4.2

ASBGo Types of Navigation: (i) Manual Mode of Operation, (ii) Autonomous Mode, and (iii) Remote Control

	Operation Modes		
Type	Manual	Autonomous	Remote control
Goals/target patients	i. Provide user's interaction with the device ii. Recommended for patients without cognitive and visual limitation and with enough motor coordination	i. Decrease the clinician burden of care ii. Clinicians may observe the patients' behavior iii. Recommended for patients with visual and cognitive impairments	i. The clinician may analyze the behavior, compensation, and changes in speed and orientations while guiding the device ii. Patients can fully focus on their rehabilitation therapy iii. Intended for patients in the initial stages of rehabilitation
Functioning	The walker is controlled by the patient considering his/her motion intention. The commands are defined on the handlebar	The clinician may set the rehabilitation scenario, indicating a target location for the walker. The walker will drive itself avoiding obstacles	The clinician commands the walker using a user-friendly and ergonomic remote control

patients during their rehabilitation therapy. It is particularly interesting since it allows the patients to fully focus on their rehabilitation therapy, without having the concern of guiding the smart walker. Moreover, the clinician is in constant observation and can support the patient if needed. In previous prototypes of ASBGo, the remote control was accomplished using a remote-control interface with a dedicated computer. The current prototype uses a small, ergonomic, and easy-to-use gamepad that sends analogic commands through Bluetooth to ASBGo's central control unit. These analogic commands are classified and translated into guidance commands, controlling the motors' speed accordingly.

Sensorial Feedback and Health Monitoring

Smart walkers should be used as therapy tools, giving support and assistance to their end-users, but also providing means of objectively quantifying the evolution of users' motor rehabilitation. Robotics-based evaluation is a major challenge in clinical practice but is necessary given the current subjective evaluation that is based on visual information and personal expertise (Moreira et al. 2019). Objective assessment, electronic records, and artificial intelligence are key technologies to attain this major challenge. This would potentiate (i) a rich stream of objective data that may assist clinicians in designing rehabilitation scenarios adjusted to each patient, (ii) a more reliable patient's diagnosis, and (iii) an objective analysis of the patient's progress throughout numerous rehabilitation sessions.

Gait and posture analyses have been important in the field of rehabilitation. Current techniques rely on expensive systems, namely Vicon (Vicon Motion Systems, UK) and Qualisys (Qualisys AB, Sweden), that need a considerable workspace and are limited to special laboratories and environments. Inertial measurement systems are also available, such as the MTw Awinda (Xsens Technologies B.V., The Netherlands), being more affordable and less environment-dependent. However, these systems require the use of markers and/or inertial sensors on the lower-limbs that, although minimally invasive, promote a lack of comfort and prohibit its use on daily life routine, thus restricting their use and access to all population (André et al. 2020).

The ASBGo Smart Walker attempts to give an affordable system for gait and posture analysis based on two embedded RGB-D cameras, as illustrated in Figure 4.2 of the "System Overview" section. Gait and posture analysis is based on a markerless and non-invasive algorithm that provides gait-specific metrics and posture assessment by tracking, respectively, the lower-limb and upper-limb. Although the proposed method is based only on depth images, the RGB image is displayed on the screen to give visual feedback to patients of their gait and posture (André et al. 2020; Caetano et al. 2016). The algorithm is based on feet and posture segmentation using standard vision-based algorithms, as illustrated in Figure 4.6.

Regarding the gait analysis, the feet position is quantified by firstly eliminating the image's background (removing the floor and walker's structure). Then, a region of interest is obtained, cropping the user's leg and some remaining inconsistencies of the floor. Afterward, the feet's contours are obtained by applying morphologic operations to the resulting image (André et al. 2020). With the feet position, it is possible to detect the gait phase (stance, swing, and double support state) and step and stride

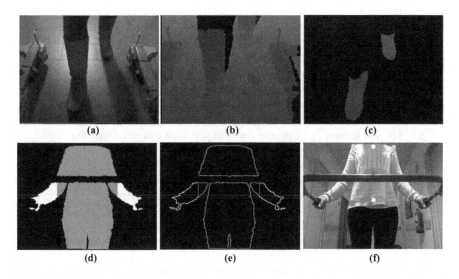

FIGURE 4.6 Feet segmentation for gait analysis: (a) RGB image with both foot, (b) depth image of both foot, (c) feet segmentation; and estimation of posture points of interest: (d) depth image with threshold, (e) contours of the torso, and (f) RGB image with points of interest. (Adapted from André et al. 2020; Caetano et al. 2016.)

transitions and calculate spatiotemporal metrics, as detailed in Table 4.3, in real time. A final session report with all the available metrics is generated and saved into the walker's database.

Regarding posture assessment, a similar algorithm is proposed to obtain the torso contours and calculate the positions of some points of interest (Caetano et al. 2016) (see Figure 4.6f). These include (i) the two iliac spine (hip) and their central point, (ii) the shoulders and their central point, and (iii) the upper-body centroid, estimating the COM's 3D position (Caetano et al. 2016). With this information, the inclination

---

TABLE 4.3

Gait-Specific Metrics Calculated with the Proposed Method Based on Depth Cameras (André et al. 2020)

	Metrics	Description
Step	Foot angle	Foot orientation at heel-strike (°)
	Width	Lateral distance between feet (cm)
	Length	Frontal displacement between the heel of the front foot when performing heel-strike and the heel of the previous foot (cm)
	Duration	Elapsed time from toe-off to heel-strike (s)
	Velocity	Displacement per unit of time (m/s)
	Cadence	Number of steps per unit of time (step/min)
Stride	Length	Displacement since heel-strike (cm)
	Duration	Elapsed time since heel-strike (s)
	Swing time	Elapsed time with the foot/leg in swing (s and % stride duration)
	Stance time	Elapsed time with the foot/leg in stance (s and % stride duration)
	Double support time	Elapsed time with both foot/leg in stance (s and % stride duration)
Global	Total distance	Distance traveled during a walking session (m)
	Total duration	Total time elapsed during a walking session (minutes)
	Average velocity	Total distance/(Total duration × 60) (m/s)
	L/R steps	Number of steps taken with the left/right foot
	L/R cadence	Average number of left/right steps per unit of time (steps/min)
	L/R distance	Total distance covered by the left/right foot (m and % total distance)
	L/R walk duration	Cumulative time of all steps taken with the left/right foot (minutes and % total duration)
	L/R average width	Average step width of both right/left foot (m)
	L/R average length	Average step length of both right/left foot (m)
	L/R step duration	Average step time elapsed for both right/left foot (s)
	L/R stride length	Average length of left/right foot strides (m)
	L/R stride duration	Average time elapsed by left/right foot strides (s)
	L/R swing duration	Average time elapsed while left/right foot is in swing (s and % of stride duration)
	L/R stance duration	Average time elapsed while left/right foot is in stance (s and % of stride duration)
	L/R double support duration	Average time elapsed while both feet are in stance (s and % of stride duration)

of the shoulders (in the axial view), the lateral inclination of the upper body (coronal view), and the frontal inclination of the body (sagittal view) are provided to the patient. This is useful to give biofeedback to patients during their therapy sessions so that they can correct their posture, enhancing their rehabilitation. Furthermore, with the COM's 3D position, the balance can be assessed by calculating the COM's velocity according to Eq. (4.1):

$$v_{COM} = \frac{\sqrt{\left(x_i - x_{i-1}\right)^2 + \left(y_i - y_{i-1}\right)^2 + \left(z_i - z_{i-1}\right)^2}}{t} \tag{4.1}$$

Results and Discussion

A benchmarking with a commercial and gold-standard motion tracker system was performed to assess the relative accuracy of the vision-based markerless gait analysis tool. Different scenarios and gait speeds were considered to attain a more extensive validation of the proposed method. The validation involved ten healthy participants and was divided into three different sessions: (i) the first session involved a conventional walker using a Vicon MX system (Vicon Motion System, UK) as ground truth, and (ii) the second session involved a treadmill walking activity with an active RGB-D camera attached to its mechanical structure. In this case, data from the force-sensing resistor and inertial system placed on each foot were used as a reference, and (iii) the third session consisted of a dynamic walk with the ASBGo Smart Walker. Each participant experienced three trials in which the gait speed varied between 0.16 and 1.0 m/s. A detailed analysis of the validation protocol is available in André et al. (2020).

The performance of the vision-based algorithm for gait analysis was assessed by comparing the measured variables with the reference systems of each session. The three trials that each participant experienced were averaged and the *root-mean-square deviation* (RMSD, in %) was computed for each session. Table 4.4 presents the main results achieved with the markerless approach. Since dimensionless measures, such as the RMSD, are dependent on the scale that is being measured, such a metric could be misleading. Therefore, metrics of Table 4.4 were also divided into

TABLE 4.4

Global, Spatial, and Temporal Performance of the Proposed Gait Analysis System When Compared to References (André et al. 2020)

	Vicon				Treadmill				Smart Walker		
Speed (m/s)	Global (%)	Spatial (cm)	Temporal (s)	Speed (m/s)	Global (%)	Spatial (cm)	Temporal (s)	Speed (m/s)	Global (%)	Spatial (cm)	Temporal (s)
0.4	35.2	5.2	0.23	0.3	57.2	15.9	1.20	0.16	50.1	3.8	0.64
0.6	44.7	4.9	0.23	0.6	30.4	14.6	0.16	0.32	31.4	6.8	0.06
1.0	58.1	6.3	0.19	0.9	30.7	15.2	0.06	0.48	30.6	6.9	0.06
				1.0	30.6	13.5	0.08	0.52	47.9	8.9	0.08

spatial (step width, step length, and stride length) and temporal (step duration, stride duration, swing time, stance time, and double support time) errors. This will allow an intuitive quantification of the proposed method's error.

The results of Table 4.4 indicate that the proposed algorithm presents a reasonable performance for temporal metrics, namely the stance, swing, and double support time, with errors lower than 0.3 s in most activities experienced. Spatial metrics, on the other side, were revealed to be not so accurate, especially for the treadmill trials. Nevertheless, the error was acceptable for the first session (with Vicon MX as reference), with errors ranging between 5 and 7 cm, and the third session (with ASBGo), with errors rounding 3–9 cm.

Regarding the posture assessment, current work is under development to assess the performance of the vision-based algorithm, performing a comparison with a commercially available MTw Awinda motion tracker system (Xsens Technologies, B.V., The Netherlands). Nevertheless, a preliminary study was conducted to assess the functionality of the system (Caetano et al. 2016). Using the points of interest calculated with the depth image of posture, ASBGo can provide visual feedback to patients so that they can correct their posture. For instance, the smart walker can recognize if the user is grabbing the handles or not and, if not, it warns the user to correctly grab the handles. Furthermore, it can also verify if the user is not having a correct posture by verifying the shoulders and torso inclination. Figure 4.7 illustrates the visual feedback the smart walker provides during a rehabilitation scenario. As illustrated in Figure 4.7, the velocity of the COM estimation is also presented, and it can be used to assess balance while walking.

Cognitive Stimulation

The inclusion of multitasking in gait training promotes faster recoveries and aids patients assimilate the gait inherently. Furthermore, due to the nature of the walk training, which is focused on the repetition of gait cycles, the development of new physiotherapy approaches is welcome to motivate patients during rehabilitation sessions. These new strategies encourage patients to perform the exercises precisely, leading to a more productive session (Yang et al. 2007). The ASBGo Smart Walker distinguishes itself from other smart walkers by also providing an interactive tool specially

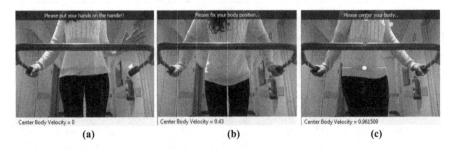

FIGURE 4.7 Visual feedback provided by the smart walker while performing posture assessment: (a) warning if the user is not grabbing the handle, and (b and c) warning if the user has a wrong posture. (Adapted from Caetano et al. 2016.)

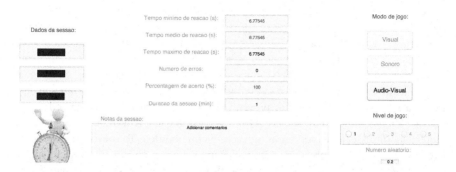

FIGURE 4.8   Multitasking game windows that display the type of game (Modo do jogo) and the results, namely the minimum/mean/maximum time of reaction (tempo mínimo/médio/ máximo de reação). Moreover, it displays the number of errors (número de erros), the accuracy (percentage de acerto), and the session duration (duração da sessão).

developed to promote a cognitive stimulation of its end-users. This tool provides several multitasking games with different operation modes. Besides the multitasking demand, the multitasking tool also assesses the end-user psychomotor condition by measuring the reaction time of the user when pressing a button in response to an external stimulus. Built in five difficulty levels for each operation mode, this game ranges from identification of a red circle in a black square to the interpretation of a sound. In other words, this tool can be adjusted to patients' skills and disabilities, allowing them to increase the difficulty of the game, as they get comfortable.

After the multitasking training session, where the patients undergo motor physiotherapy with the smart walker while playing the game, a final window appears with the performance results, as illustrated in Figure 4.8. These data include the minimum, maximum, and average of the reaction times of the player, the number of errors, the accuracy of their responses, and the duration of the session. The results can be used by the medical staff to evaluate the patient's mental requesting.

Safety Mechanisms

As mentioned in the introduction of this chapter, more than 30% of users stop using their assistive devices because they do not feel confident with them or because these assistive devices are not particularly suited for them (Bateni and Maki 2005). By following since early a user-oriented design, the ASBGo Smart Walker provides different mechanisms to ensure the safety of its end-users.

The navigation system mode includes obstacle detection and avoidance functionality using the embedded ultrasonic sensors (Moreira et al. 2019; Faria et al. 2014). These sensors are useful to detect potential collisions with punctual obstacles that could lead to the user's instability, resulting in an increased risk of falls. This functionality is currently being improved in the fourth prototype to ensure safe therapies that augment the user's confidence and willingness to use the product. As discussed earlier in the "Navigation Assistance" section, a laser range finder is used to map the environment and detect permanent and/or punctual obstacles. This improvement makes ASBGo an environment context-aware smart walker.

Another safety mechanism provided by ASBGo is an emergency button. This safety mechanism is particularly important since, when the button is pressed, it immediately stops the walker. This emergency button is directly connected to the motors' power supply and can be activated whenever the user loses control over ASBGo, increasing the risk of fall, or in a sudden event of system failure, for instance.

The team is also developing a safety mechanism that predicts a near-fall and stops the smart walker immediately to prevent major consequences. As discussed earlier, falls are a major concern for society. They may result in death or in several injuries that require motor assistance, representing an economic burden. To overcome these problems, a diversity of fall prevention strategies implemented on assistive devices such as smart walkers have been widely explored. When smart walkers detect situations that may lead to a fall, they usually stop providing support to the user (Pereira, Ribeiro, and Santos 2019). Current fall prevention strategies usually require information from non-wearable sensors placed on the walker, e.g., laser range finders (LRF) (Xu, Huang, and Cheng 2018), stereo cameras (Taghvaei, Hirata, and Kosuge 2010), force/torque sensors (Xu, Huang, and Cheng 2018), and depth cameras (Taghvaei and Kosuge 2018).

Before implementing the near-fall detection in ASBGo, the team decided to investigate what information is important to detect near-falls in a conventional rollator. Toward a minimal sensor setup and computational load for real-time application, the approach is based on an IMU placed at the user's sacrum along with FSRs on both feet. These sensors have already been studied for predicting near-falls, as mentioned in Taghvaei and Kosuge (2018), but without the support of any rollator. Figure 4.9 illustrates the system description to predict near-fall detection.

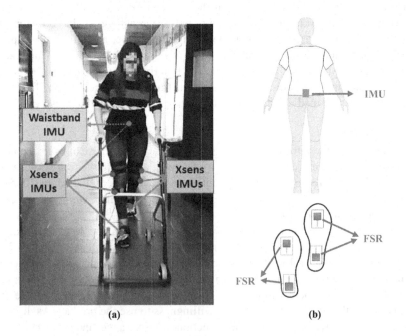

(a)   (b)

FIGURE 4.9 System description: (a) waistband IMU and rollator and (b) wearable sensors location (IMU – on the user's sacrum, FSR – on the heel and toe).

The information gathered with both sensors, i.e., IMU and FSRs, is used to compute several features that will act as inputs for machine learning classifiers. In this work, the team studied the use of several machine-learning classifiers, namely discriminant analysis, K-nearest neighbors – KNN, ensemble learning, decision tree – DT, and support vector machine. Nearly 170 features were computed, as described in Table 4.5, but not all were used in the near-fall detection. Three feature selection algorithms were used to rank the 60 most important features, namely the minimum-redundancy-maximum-relevancy (mRMR), the Relief-F, and the principal component analysis (PCA).

TABLE 4.5
Feature Description. The Most Important Features Found with the mRMR Feature Selection Method are Highlighted in Bold

Feature Description

Acceleration – Acc (V, **ML**, **AP**), angular velocity – Gyr (V, **ML**, AP); 4 FSR signals: **toe right**, heel right, toe left, and heel left.

Sum vector magnitude (SumVM) of Acc and Gyr[a]

Skewness, kurtosis, **minimum**, maximum (**AP**), **mean**, variance, standard deviation of Acc – (V, ML, AP)

Skewness, kurtosis, **minimum**, maximum (**ML**), mean (**ML**), variance, standard deviation of Gyr – (V, ML, AP)

Skewness, kurtosis, **minimum**, maximum (**Gyr**), **mean**, variance, standard deviation of SumVM of Acc and Gyr

Correlation between axes – Acc and Gyr – (V-ML, V-AP, ML-AP)

Acc after high-pass filter (**AP**, ML, **V**)[b]

SumVM of Acc raw data[a], dynamic sum vector[a], vertical Acc[a], **total angular change**, resultant angular Acc[b], activity signal magnitude area (ASMA)[b], signal magnitude area (SMA)

Peak-to-peak values (PPV), root mean square (RMS) (**AP**), ratio index (RI), RI of PPV of Acc – (V, ML, AP)

PPV, RMS (**V**, **AP**), RI, RI of PPV of Gyr – (V, ML, AP)

PPV, RMS, RI, RI of PPV of SumVM of Acc and Gyr

Quaternions[b], Roll[b], Pitch[b], Yaw[b], and **absolute vertical Acc**[a]

SumVM of resultant angle change[a], maximum resultant angular acceleration, Sum of fluctuation frequency, **SumVM of resultant of average Acc**[a], **SumVM of resultant of standard deviation**[a]

Resultant angle change[b], fluctuation frequency, resultant of average Acc[b] (**AP**, **ML**), resultant of standard deviation[b] (**AP**, **ML**), gravity component[a], velocity (**AP**, **V**), displacement (**AP**, **V**), **cumulative horizontal sway length**, mean sway velocity (**ML**, **V**), **displacement range** – (AP, ML, V)

Slope[b], fast change vector, SumVM of horizontal plane[a], EMA[b], rotational angle using Acc[b], **Z-score**[a], magnitude of angular displacement[a], Acc and Gyr resultant of delta changes[b], cumulative horizontal displacement

[a] *Features that require only the current sample from initial data;*
[b] *Features that require only the current and the previous samples from initial data;*
Except the first ten features, the remaining features require a time-window of five samples (current sample and the four previous ones).
V: vertical; ML: mediolateral; AP: anteroposterior.

Results and Discussion

To predict a near-fall detection, a data collection involving 10 able-bodied participants (5 females and 5 males; 25 ± 1.61 years old, 1.69 ± 0.11 m, and 66.5 ± 11.3 kg)
was conducted. The participants walked with the support of a conventional rollator
(see Figure 4.9) for four different activities at two different gait speeds (comfortable
and slow): (i) walk forward for 10 m and (ii) walk forward and simulate near-falls
to the right, left, and forward. This resulted in 240 trials of which 180 included
near-falls.

After data collection, data were filtered, and the features of Table 4.5 were calculated. They were normalized by the user's body height and scaled between 0 and
1 with a maximum-minimum algorithm. For machine learning purposes, data were
split within the training and test dataset following a holdout method. Moreover, data
were labeled within two classes with a binary target: 0 corresponds to normal walk
and 1 corresponds to a near-fall detection. The performance was evaluated by calculating the accuracy, sensitivity, specificity, precision, $F1$-score, and Matthews correlation coefficient (MCC). Figure 4.10 illustrates the overview of the different steps
performed to discriminate the near-fall from normal walking.

From these procedures, the team identified the Ensemble Learning with the first
51 features ranked by the mRMR as the most accurate machine learning classifier for
near-fall detection while using test data. The best model yields an accuracy of 95.2%,
a precision of 94.9%, a sensitivity of 71.6%, a specificity of 99.3%, an $F1$-score of
81.7%, and an MCC of 79.9%, with the following hyperparameters: (i) ensemble
aggregation method – bag; (ii) learning cycles – 498; (iii) minimum leaf size – 1; and
(iv) no learn rate. A post-processing method based on a time window that contains
the current and past classifier outputs was performed to increase the strategy performance. When using test data, a near-fall was detected on average 0.71 ± 0.48 s after
the start and 1.48 ± 0.68 s before the recovery, being able to detect all 56 near-falls
from test data. The number of misclassified normal walking samples decreased by
98%. These results show that the proposed strategy accurately detects a near-fall,
which is important to provide the safety of the end-user when using the ASBGo
Smart Walker.

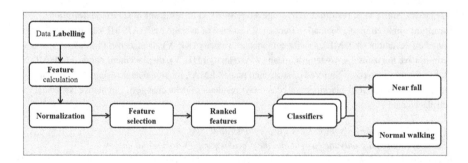

FIGURE 4.10 Schematic overview of the different steps performed to discriminate the near-
fall detection from normal walking.

CLINICAL EVALUATION

Evidence suggests that individuals with ataxia may benefit from the motor and functional long-term training. After intensive treatments in this area, patients with cerebellar disorders have shown improvement in motor and functional tasks (Martins, Santos, et al. 2015). The ASBGo Smart Walker was specifically designed to adapt to the ataxic patients' needs, intended to aid them in regaining their independence and improving their quality of life. Since patients present different necessities according to their intrinsic characteristics, ASBGo can provide different functionalities, enhancing its effectiveness as a rehabilitation tool. Clinical evaluations were carried out with previous prototypes of ASBGo, enabling to quantify the gait evolution and to identify the problems that benefited from this treatment, as well as the best outcome measures. In this chapter, the main results achieved will be presented. A detailed analysis of the smart walker clinical evaluation is available in Martins (2015).

Cases of Study

The clinical study involved three cases of study: (i) Patient 1 is a 64-year-old male. In 2014, he presented with sudden right ataxic hemiparesis, due to neurobrucellosis. He started antibiotic therapy and rehabilitation program. At the beginning of the therapy, he scored 6/56 points on the Berg balance scale (BBS) and required the assistance of two people to walk. (ii) Patient 2 is a 28-year-old female, with cerebellar pilocytic astrocytoma, surgically removed in 2005. She presented gait ataxia, dysarthria, nystagmus, bilateral upper limb dysmetria, and intention tremor. She did not show significant improvement since the recovery period after surgery, even though doing physiotherapy regularly. She scored 12/56 on BBS and was able to walk with two crutches, but with close supervision of a third person. (iii) Patient 3 is a 46-year-old female, with ataxic tetraparesis and lesion of cranial nerves VI, VII, IX, and X, due to a petroclival meningioma surgically removed in 11/2014. She underwent surgical tracheostomy and percutaneous endoscopic gastrostomy. She was not able to sit and stand-alone or walk without the help of a third person. She scored 4/56 on BBS and required assistance to stand and walk.

Intervention

Regarding Patient 1, he was trained with the Smart Walker for three weeks, 5 days a week. He was able to drive the walker itself. Velocity was set by the clinician and the first sessions were set to last for 15 minutes. Such velocity and time were increased when the patient felt comfortable doing so.

Patient 2 was trained assisted gait with the smart walker twice a week, performing a total of 40 sessions (eight weeks). The first 20 sessions were performed also with aquatic therapy and the last 20 sessions were performed only with the smart walker. In the first five sessions, the remote control was used to guide the walker, since the patient was not capable to concentrate on guiding at the same time she corrected her gait pattern. Then, since she already had enough cognitive capacity to guide the walker, she handled such a task. Velocity was set by the physiotherapist and the first sessions were set to last for 15 minutes.

At last, Patient 3 was submitted to conventional physiotherapy for 20 sessions (four weeks). After these sessions, the smart walker was added to her therapy. During the first ten sessions (2 weeks) with the smart walker, the remote control was used. In the remaining 6 weeks, manual guidance was set since the patient was already capable of handling such a task. Velocity was set by the physiotherapist and the first sessions were set to last for 10 minutes.

Spatiotemporal Gait Parameters

Each patient was evaluated by calculating step and stride length (STP and STR, respectively), stride width (WIDTH), gait cycle (GC), cadence (CAD), velocity (VEL), stance and swing phase duration (STAD and SWD, respectively), double support duration (DS), and step time (STPT). With this information, symmetry indices (SI) were calculated for each feature using Eq (4.2), where U_R and U_L are, respectively, the features for both right (R) and left (L) legs. Perfect symmetry results if SI is zero, larger positive and negative deviations would indicate a greater symmetry toward the right or left leg, respectively. This chapter will present the main conclusions regarding the SI for all calculated features. Further results are available in Martins (2015).

$$\text{Symmetry index } = \frac{U_R - U_L}{U_L} \qquad (4.2)$$

Postural Stability

Postural stability was assessed with an accelerometer located near the COM, at the level of the sacrum. Each patient was evaluated in both static and dynamic positions. A static position was performed without the smart walker, and a dynamic position was assessed while the users were walking with the smart walker. The calculated postural stability parameters are the *root-mean-square* of anteroposterior (AP), horizontal (HOR), and mediolateral (ML) accelerations (RMSAP, RMSHOR, and RMSML), range of motion of AP and ML directions (ROMAP and ROMML), and sway length (SLML, SLAP, and SLHOR). Additionally, the COM trajectory in AP and ML directions was also acquired. This chapter will present the main results regarding the COM trajectory considering the AP and ML directions. Further results are available in Martins (2015).

Results and Discussion

Figure 4.11 presents the symmetry index for the three cases of study: (a) Patient 1, (b) Patient 2, and (c) Patient 3, regarding the gait-specific metrics that were assessed in this clinical evaluation. By analyzing Figure 4.11, all patients exhibited an asymmetrical gait at the beginning of the clinical trials since a symmetry index different from zero was obtained. Although not presenting a high value of symmetry index, the patients exhibit a stumble and unstable walk. However, throughout the therapy sessions, a decrease was verified in the patients' symmetry index, tending toward a near-zero value. These results show that, indeed, the smart walker helped the patients' gait recovery since, at the end of the therapy, they all showed improvements

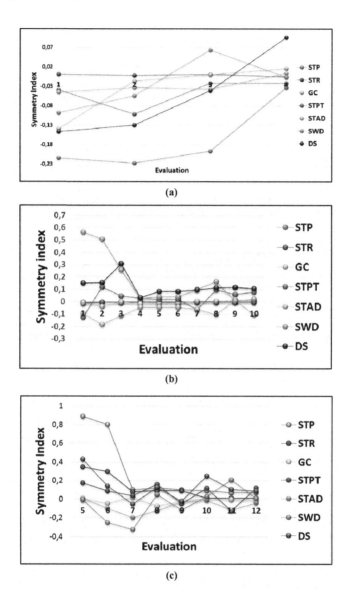

FIGURE 4.11 Symmetry index for the three cases of study while walking with the smart walker.

in the STP, STR, GC, STPT, STAD, SWD, and DS, with similar values for both right and left legs.

Considering the postural assessment, the three patients also experienced an improvement in the COM trajectory considering the anteroposterior and mediolateral displacements. Figure 4.12 illustrates the COM variation considering AP and ML displacements considering: (a) Patient 1, (b) Patient 2, and (c) Patient 3, and considering both static (comfortable stance) and dynamic balance (with the smart walker).

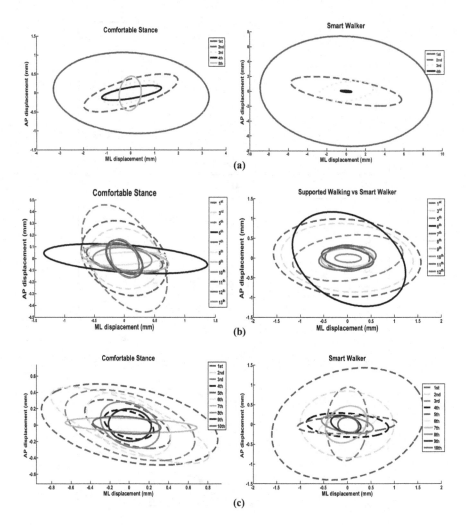

FIGURE 4.12 COM trajectory for the three cases of study considering AP and ML displacements.

Moreover, COM displacement is depicted for all the training sessions that each patient experienced with the smart walker.

By analyzing Figure 4.12, all patients present high AP and ML displacements in the first sessions. Also, it is visible that all patients present a higher ML displacement in comparison with the AP displacement, which increased their tendency to fall sideways. This is a typical symptom of ataxic patients since they often exhibit a lack of motor coordination, poor balance, and, thus, less equilibrium. However, throughout the sessions with the smart walker, the ellipse-shaped COM displacement improved, especially the ML displacement that improved considerably when compared with the first sessions. Moreover, patients also improved their static balance, which is evaluated without any support provided by the smart walker. This is a positive result since it shows that patients regain their balance coordination, which is of utmost importance to improve their gait and decrease the risk of falls.

The intensity-adapted gait training and the physical support given by ASBGo boosted the patients' balance and motor coordination, improving both gait and postural control. The patients regain a part of their motor functionalities, enhancing their residual motor skills. This was accomplished by fostering a user-oriented therapy, considering since early the patients' clinical needs. By providing intensity-adapted, personalized, and user-oriented assistance, the ASBGo smart walker proved to be an important rehabilitation tool. Further clinical evaluations are being considered with the current prototype, performing a longitudinal study with more ataxic patients to revalidate all the algorithms and functionalities that are presented in this chapter.

CONCLUSIONS

This chapter presents the importance of smart walkers in biomedical robotic technologies and healthcare engineering. An overview of current smart walkers on literature was presented, with their main advantages and limitations over conventional walkers and rehabilitation therapies. The ASBGo Smart Walker was also presented. Its mechanical structure, architecture, main functionalities, and clinical evaluation were presented and detailed. ASBGo is a personalized and user-oriented assistive device that acts as a rehabilitation tool for ataxic gait and posture rehabilitation, fostering human–robot interaction that encourages users to actively participate in the rehabilitation therapies, enhancing their residual motor skills. Its embedded sensors, namely force sensors, RGB-D cameras, lasers, and sonars, allow the end-users' continuous health monitoring by assessing and monitoring gait-specific and posture parameters while ensuring their safety with navigation assistance and obstacle avoidance. Furthermore, visual feedback of gait and posture is provided to allow a self-correction, augmenting the chances of effective rehabilitation. The walker is also controlled remotely, which can be useful to clinicians to observe the patients' rehabilitation and reactions to external stimuli. Additionally, the walker provides a multitasking tool with different types of games and levels to provide the patients cognitive stimulus, enhancing their neurological recovery as well. At last, the smart walker proved to be clinically relevant by improving the patients' gait with symmetry indexes near-zero (thus, indicating an improvement in the gait symmetry) and in the posture with smaller center-of-mass displacements regarding anteroposterior and mediolateral planes. Future work will address more experimental studies with ataxic patients to continuously assess the walker's benefit in gait and posture rehabilitation.

ACKNOWLEDGMENTS

This research has been supported in part by FEDER Funds through COMPETE 2020 – Programa Operacional Competitividade e Internacionalização (POCI) and P2020 with the Reference Project EML under Grant POCI-01–0247-FEDER-033067, and by FCT national funds, under the national support to R&D units grant, through the reference project UIDB/04436/2020 and UIDP/04436/2020, and with the scholarship reference PD/BD/141515/2018.

REFERENCES

Alves, Joana, Eurico Seabra, Inês Caetano, José Gonçalves, João Serra, Maria Martins, and Cristina P. Santos. 2016. "Considerations and Mechanical Modifications on a Smart Walker." In *Proceedings – 2016 International Conference on Autonomous Robot Systems and Competitions, ICARSC 2016*, 247–52. doi:10.1109/ICARSC.2016.30.

André, João, João M. Lopes, Manuel Palermo, Diogo Gonçalves, Ana Matias, Fátima Pereira, José Afonso, Eurico Seabra, João Cerqueira, and Cristina P. Santos. 2020. "Markerless Gait Analysis Vision System for Real-Time Gait Monitoring." In *2020 IEEE International Conference on Autonomous Robot Systems and Competitions*, 269–74, Ponta Delgada, Portugal.

Annicchiarico, Roberta, Cristian Barrué, T. Benedico, Fabio Campana, Ulises Cortés, and Antonio Martínez-Velasco. 2008. "The I-Walker: An Intelligent Pedestrian Mobility Aid." *Frontiers in Artificial Intelligence and Applications* 178: 708–12. doi:10.3233/978-1-58603-891-5-708.

Barbeau, Hugues, and Martha Visintin. 2003. "Optimal Outcomes Obtained With Body-Weight Support Combined With Treadmill Training in Stroke Subjects." *Archives of Physical Medicine and Rehabilitation* 84 (10): 1458–65. doi:10.1053/S0003-9993(03)00361-7.

Bateni, Hamid, and Brian E. Maki. 2005. "Assistive Devices for Balance and Mobility: Benefits, Demands, and Adverse Consequences." *Archives of Physical Medicine and Rehabilitation* 86 (1): 134–45. doi:10.1016/j.apmr.2004.04.023.

Beckerle, Philipp, Gionata Salvietti, Ramazan Unal, Domenico Prattichizzo, Simone Rossi, Claudio Castellini, Hirche Sandra, Satoshi Endo, Heni Ben Amor, Matei Ciocarlie, Fulvio Mastrogiovanni, Breena D. Argall, and Matteo Bianchi. 2017. "A Human-Robot Interaction Perspective on Assistive and Rehabilitation Robotics." *Frontiers in Neurorobotics* 11 (May): 1–6. doi:10.3389/fnbot.2017.00024.

Berg, Katherine Olga, Sharon L. Wood-Dauphinee, Jackson Ivan Williams, and Brian Edward Maki. 1992. "Measuring Balance in the Elderly: Validation of an Instrument." *Canadian Journal of Public Health* 83 (Suppl. 2): S7–11.

Bradley, Sara M., and Cameron R. Hernandez. 2011. "Geriatric Assistive Devices." *American Family Physician* 84 (4): 405–11.

Buckley, Ellen, Claudia Mazzà, and Alisdair McNeill. 2018. "A Systematic Review of the Gait Characteristics Associated with Cerebellar Ataxia." *Gait and Posture* 60 (November 2017): 154–63. doi:10.1016/j.gaitpost.2017.11.024.

Caetano, Inês, Joana Alves, José Gonçalves, Maria Martins, and Cristina P. Santos. 2016. "Development of a Biofeedback Approach Using Body Tracking with Active Depth Sensor in ASBGo Smart Walker." In *Proceedings – 2016 International Conference on Autonomous Robot Systems and Competitions, ICARSC 2016*, 241–46. doi:10.1109/ICARSC.2016.34.

Chang, Ming Fang, Wei Hao Mou, Chien Ke Liao, and Li Chen Fu. 2012. "Design and Implementation of an Active Robotic Walker for Parkinson's Patients." In *Proceedings of the SICE Annual Conference*. IEEE, 2068–73, Akita, Japan.

Cifuentes, Carlos A., Camilo Rodriguez, Anselmo Frizera-Neto, Teodiano Freire Bastos-Filho, and Ricardo Carelli. 2016. "Multimodal Human–Robot Interaction for Walker-Assisted Gait." *IEEE Systems Journal* 10 (3): 933–43. doi:10.1109/JSYST.2014.2318698.

Cortés, Ulisses, Antonio Martínez-Velasco, Cristian Barrué, Estefanía Martín, Fabio Campana, Roberta Annicchiarico, and Carlo Caltagirone. 2008. "Towards an Intelligent Service to Elders Mobility Using the I-Walker." *AAAI Fall Symposium – Technical Report* FS-08-02 (August 2014): 32–38.

Efthimiou, Eleni, Stavroula-Evita Fotinea, Theodore Goulas, Athanasia-Lida Dimou, Maria Koutsombogera, Vassilis Pitsikalis, Petros Maragos, and Costas Tzafestas. 2016. "The MOBOT Platform – Showcasing Multimodality in Human-Assistive Robot Interaction." In *Lecture Notes in Computer Science*. Springer, Cham.

Faria, Vitor, Jorge Silva, Maria Martins, and Cristina Santos. 2014. "Dynamical System Approach for Obstacle Avoidance in a Smart Walker Device." *2014 IEEE International Conference on Autonomous Robot Systems and Competitions, ICARSC 2014*. IEEE, 261–66. doi:10.1109/ICARSC.2014.6849796.

Ferrari, Francesco, Stefano Divan, Cristina Guerrero, Fabiano Zenatti, Roberta Guidolin, Luigi Palopoli, and Daniele Fontanelli. 2020. "Human–Robot Interaction Analysis for a Smart Walker for Elderly: The ACANTO Interactive Guidance System." *International Journal of Social Robotics* 12 (2): 479–92. doi:10.1007/s12369-019-00572-5.

Fonteyn, Ella M. R., Tanja Schmitz-Hübsch, Carla C. Verstappen, Laslo Baliko, Bastiaan R. Bloem, Silvia Boesch, Lisa Bunn, Perrine Charles, Alexandra Dürr, Alessandro Filla, Paola Giunti, Christoph Globas, Thomas Klockgether, Bela Melegh, Massimo Pandolfo, Anna De Rosa, Ludger Schöls, Dagmar Timmann, Marten Munneke, Berry P. H. Kremer, and Bart P. C. Van De Warrenburg 2010. "Falls in Spinocerebellar Ataxias: Results of the EuroSCA Fall Study." *Cerebellum* 9 (2): 232–39. doi:10.1007/s12311-010-0155-z.

Frizera-Neto, Anselmo, Ramón Ceres, Eduardo Rocon, and José Luis Pons. 2011. "Empowering and Assisting Natural Human Mobility: The Simbiosis Walker." *International Journal of Advanced Robotic Systems* 8 (3): 34–50. doi:10.5772/10666.

Gelder, Linda M. A. van, Andrew Barnes, Jonathan S. Wheat, and Ben W. Heller. 2018. "The Use of Biofeedback for Gait Retraining: A Mapping Review." *Clinical Biomechanics* 59 (September): 159–66. doi:10.1016/j.clinbiomech.2018.09.020.

Giggins, Oonagh M., Ulrik McCarthy Persson, and Brian Caulfield. 2013. "Biofeedback in Rehabilitation." *Journal of NeuroEngineering and Rehabilitation* 10 (60). doi:10.1007/978-1-4899-3083-5_5.

Huang, Cunjun, Glenn Wasson, Majd Alwan, Pradip Sheth, and Alexandre Ledoux. 2005. "Shared Navigational Control and User Intent Detection in an Intelligent Walker." *AAAI Fall Symposium – Technical Report* FS-05-02: 59–66.

Huang, Jian, Wenxia Xu, Samer Mohammed, and Zhen Shu. 2015. "Posture Estimation and Human Support Using Wearable Sensors and Walking-Aid Robot." *Robotics and Autonomous Systems* 73: 24–43. doi:10.1016/j.robot.2014.11.013.

Ilg, Winfried, Heidrun Golla, Peter Thier, and Martin A. Giese. 2007. "Specific Influences of Cerebellar Dysfunctions on Gait." *Brain* 130 (3): 786–98. doi:10.1093/brain/awl376.

Ilg, Winfried, and Dagmar Timmann. 2013. "Gait Ataxia-Specific Cerebellar Influences and Their Rehabilitation." *Movement Disorders* 28 (11): 1566–75. doi:10.1002/mds.25558.

Jiménez, Mario F., Matias Monllor, Anselmo Frizera, Teodiano Bastos, Flavio Roberti, and Ricardo Carelli. 2019. "Admittance Controller with Spatial Modulation for Assisted Locomotion Using a Smart Walker." *Journal of Intelligent and Robotic Systems: Theory and Applications* 94 (3–4): 621–37. doi:10.1007/s10846-018-0854-0.

Lacey, Gerard J., and Diego Rodriguez-Losada. 2008. "A Smart Walker for the Blind." *Robotics & Automation Magazine*, no. December: 75–83.

Lee, Geunho, Eui Jung Jung, Takanori Ohnuma, Nak Young Chong, and Byung Ju Yi. 2011. "JAIST Robotic Walker Control Based on a Two-Layered Kalman Filter." *Proceedings – IEEE International Conference on Robotics and Automation*. IEEE, 3682–87. doi:10.1109/ICRA.2011.5979784.

Lee, Geunho, Takanori Ohnuma, and Nak Young Chong. 2010. "Design and Control of JAIST Active Robotic Walker." *Intelligent Service Robotics* 3 (3): 125–35. doi:10.1007/s11370-010-0064-5.

Lim, Chung Dial, Chia Ming Wang, Ching Ying Cheng, Yen Chao, Shih Huan Tseng, and Li Chen Fu. 2016. "Sensory Cues Guided Rehabilitation Robotic Walker Realized by Depth Image-Based Gait Analysis." *IEEE Transactions on Automation Science and Engineering* 13 (1): 171–80. doi:10.1109/TASE.2015.2494067.

Martins, Maria. 2015. "ASBGo: A Smart Walker for Mobility Assistance and Monitoring System Aid." Doctoral thesis presented to the University of Minho.

Martins, Maria, Vitor Faria, Jorge Silva, and Cristina P. Santos. 2015. "Autonomous Mode Experiments." https://www.youtube.com/watch?v=wfmFeA60B0o&feature=youtu.be.

Martins, Maria M., Cristina P. Santos, Anselmo Frizera-Neto, and Ramn Ceres. 2012. "Assistive Mobility Devices Focusing on Smart Walkers: Classification and Review." *Robotics and Autonomous Systems* 60 (4): 548–62. doi:10.1016/j.robot.2011.11.015.

Martins, Maria, Cristina Santos, and Anselmo Frizera. 2012. "Online Control of a Mobility Assistance Smart Walker." In *2012 IEEE 2nd Portuguese Meeting in Bioengineering, ENBENG 2012.* IEEE. doi:10.1109/ENBENG.2012.6331388.

Martins, Maria, Cristina P. Santos, Anselmo Frizera, Ana Matias, Tania Pereira, Maria Cotter, and Fatima Pereira. 2015. "Smart Walker Use for Ataxia's Rehabilitation: Case Study." In *IEEE International Conference on Rehabilitation Robotics* 2015 September, 852–57. doi:10.1109/ICORR.2015.7281309.

Martins, Maria, Cristina P. Santos, Eurico Seabra, Anselmo Frizera, and Ramón Ceres. 2014. "Design, Implementation and Testing of a New User Interface for a Smart Walker." *2014 IEEE International Conference on Autonomous Robot Systems and Competitions, ICARSC 2014,* 217–22. doi:10.1109/ICARSC.2014.6849789.

Meng, Wei, Quan Liu, Zude Zhou, Qingsong Ai, Bo Sheng, and Shengquan Shane Xie. 2015. "Recent Development of Mechanisms and Control Strategies for Robot-Assisted Lower Limb Rehabilitation." *Mechatronics* 31: 132–45. doi:10.1016/j. mechatronics.2015.04.005.

Mikolajczyk, Tadeusz, Ileana Ciobanu, Doina Ioana Badea, Alina Iliescu, Sara Pizzamiglio, Thomas Schauer, Thomas Seel, Petre Lucian Seiciu, Duncan L. Turner, and Mihai Berteanu. 2018. "Advanced Technology for Gait Rehabilitation: An Overview." *Advances in Mechanical Engineering* 10 (7): 1–19. doi:10.1177/1687814018783627.

Milne, Sarah C., Louise A. Corben, Nellie Georgiou-Karistianis, Martin B. Delatycki, and Eppie M. Yiu. 2017. "Rehabilitation for Individuals with Genetic Degenerative Ataxia: A Systematic Review." *Neurorehabilitation and Neural Repair* 31 (7): 609–22. doi:10.1177/1545968317712469.

Moreira, Rui, Joana Alves, Ana Matias, and Cristina P. Santos. 2019. "Smart and Assistive Walker – ASBGo: Rehabilitation Robotics: A Smart-Walker to Assist Ataxic Patients." In *Robotics in Healthcare. Advances in Experimental Medicine and Biology,* edited by J. Siqueira, 37–68. Springer Nature. doi:10.1007/978-3-319-32669-6.

Mun, Kyung Ryoul, Su Bin Lim, Zhao Guo, and Haoyong Yu. 2017. "Biomechanical Effects of Body Weight Support with a Novel Robotic Walker for Over-Ground Gait Rehabilitation." *Medical and Biological Engineering and Computing* 55 (2): 315–26. doi:10.1007/s11517-016-1515-8.

Neto, Anselmo Frizera, Arlindo Elias, Carlos Cifuentes, Camilo Rodriguez, Teodiano Bastos, and Ricardo Carelli. 2015. "Smart Walkers: Advanced Robotic Human Walking-Aid Systems." *Intelligent Assistive Robots* 106: 103–31. doi:10.1007/978-3-319-12922-8.

Paulo, João. 2017. "A Multimodal HMI Approach for Interaction, User Modeling and Automatic Gait Analysis on a Robotic Walker." Doctoral thesis presented to University of Coimbra, Portugal.

Paulo, João, Paulo Peixoto, and Urbano J. Nunes. 2017. "ISR-AIWALKER: Robotic Walker for Intuitive and Safe Mobility Assistance and Gait Analysis." *IEEE Transactions on Human-Machine Systems* 47 (6): 1110–22. doi:10.1109/THMS.2017.2759807.

Pereira, António, Nuno F. Ribeiro, and Cristina P. Santos. 2019. "A Survey of Fall Prevention Systems Implemented on Smart Walkers *." In *2019 IEEE 6th Portuguese Meeting on Bioengineering (ENBENG),* 1–4. doi:10.1109/ENBENG.2019.8692530.

Rentschler, Andrew J., Richard Simpson, Rory A. Cooper, and Michael L. Boninger. 2008. "Clinical Evaluation of Guido Robotic Walker." *Journal of Rehabilitation Research and Development* 45 (9): 1281–94. doi:10.1682/JRRD.2007.10.0160.

Schmitz-Hübsch, Tanja, Sophie Tezenas Du Montcel, László Baliko, José A. Berciano, Sylvia M. Boesch, Chantal Depondt, Paola Giunti, Christoph Globas, Jon Infante, Jun-suk Kang, Berry P. H. Kremer, Caterina Mariotti, Béla I. Melegh, Massimo Pandolfo, Maria J. Rakowicz, Pascale Ribai, Rafal X. Rola, Lüdger Schöls, Sandra Szymanski, Bart P. C. Van Du Warrenburg, Alexandra Dürr, Thomas Klockgether, and Roberto Fancellu. 2006. "Scale for the Assessment and Rating of Ataxia: Development of a New Clinical Scale." *Neurology* 66 (11): 1717–20. doi:10.1212/01.wnl.0000219042.60538.92.
Sierra, Sergio D., Mario Garzón, Marcela Múnera, and Carlos A. Cifuentes. 2019. "Human–Robot–Environment Interaction Interface for Smart Walker Assisted Gait: AGoRA Walker." *Sensors (Switzerland)* 19 (13): 1–29. doi:10.3390/s19132897.
Sierra, Sergio D., Juan F. Molina, Daniel A. Gomez, Marcela C. Munera, and Carlos A. Cifuentes. 2018. "Development of an Interface for Human-Robot Interaction on a Robotic Platform for Gait Assistance: AGoRA Smart Walker." *2018 IEEE ANDESCON, ANDESCON 2018 – Conference Proceedings*. IEEE. doi:10.1109/ANDESCON.2018.8564594.
Silva, Jorge, Cristina P. Santos, and João Sequeira. 2013. "Navigation Architecture for Mobile Robots with Temporal Stabilization of Movements." In *9th International Workshop on Robot Motion and Control, RoMoCo 2013 – Workshop Proceedings*, 209–14. doi:10.1109/RoMoCo.2013.6614610.
Spenko, Matthew, Haoyong Yu, and Steven Dubowsky. 2006. "Robotic Personal Aids for Mobility and Monitoring for the Elderly." *IEEE Transactions on Neural Systems and Rehabilitation Engineering* 14 (3): 344–51. doi:10.1109/TNSRE.2006.881534.
Stanton, Rosalyn, Louise Ada, Catherine M. Dean, and Elisabeth Preston. 2017. "Biofeedback Improves Performance in Lower Limb Activities More than Usual Therapy in People Following Stroke: A Systematic Review." *Journal of Physiotherapy* 63 (1): 11–16. doi:10.1016/j.jphys.2016.11.006.
Taghvaei, Sajjad, Yuuichi Hirata, and Kazuhiro Kosuge. 2010. "Vision-Based Human State Estimation to Control an Intelligent Passive Walker." In *2010 IEEE/SICE International Symposium on System Integration*, 146–51. doi:10.1109/SII.2010.5708316.
Taghvaei, Sajjad, and Kazuhiro Kosuge. 2018. "Image-Based Fall Detection and Classification of a User with a Walking Support System." *Frontiers of Mechanical Engineering* 13 (3): 427–41. doi:10.1007/s11465-017-0465-7.
Tercero-Pérez, Karla, Hernán Cortés, Yessica Torres-Ramos, Roberto Rodríguez-Labrada, César M. Cerecedo-Zapata, Oscar Hernández-Hernández, Nelson Pérez-González, Rigoberto González-Piña, Norberto Leyva-García, Bulmaro Cisneros, Luis Velázquez-Pérez, and Jonathan J. Magaña. 2019. "Effects of Physical Rehabilitation in Patients with Spinocerebellar Ataxia Type 7." *Cerebellum* 18 (3): 397–405. doi:10.1007/s12311-019-1006-1.
Tucker, Michael R., Olivier Lambercy, Roger Gassert, Jeremy Olivier, Hannes Bleuler, Mohamed Bouri, Anna Pagel, Robert Riener, Heike Vallery, and José R. Del Millán. 2015. "Control Strategies for Active Lower Extremity Prosthetics and Orthotics: A Review." *Journal of NeuroEngineering and Rehabilitation* 12 (1). doi:10.1186/1743-0003-12-1.
World Health Organization. 2011a. "Disability – a global picture", in *World Report on Disability*: 19–54.
World Health Organization. 2011b. "Rehabilitation." In *World Report on Disability*: 93–134.
Xu, Wenxia, Jian Huang, and Lei Cheng. 2018. "A Novel Coordinated Motion Fusion-Based Walking-Aid Robot System." *Sensors* 18 (9). doi:10.3390/s18092761.
Yang, Yea Ru, Ray Yau Wang, Yu Chung Chen, and Mu Jung Kao. 2007. "Dual-Task Exercise Improves Walking Ability in Chronic Stroke: A Randomized Controlled Trial." *Archives of Physical Medicine and Rehabilitation* 88 (10): 1236–40. doi:10.1016/j.apmr.2007.06.762.

Ye, Jianyu, Jian Huang, Jiping He, Chunjing Tao, and Xitai Wang. 2012. "Development of a Width-Changeable Intelligent Walking-Aid Robot." *2012 International Symposium on Micro-NanoMechatronics and Human Science (MHS)*. IEEE, 358–63, Nagoya, Japan.

Ye, Jing, Gong Chen, Quanquan Liu, Lihong Duan, Wanfeng Shang, Xifan Yao, Jianjun Long, Yulong Wang, Zhengzhi Wu, and Chunbao Wang. 2018. "An Adaptive Shared Control of a Novel Robotic Walker for Gait Rehabilitation of Stroke Patients." *2018 International Conference on Intelligence and Safety for Robotics, ISR 2018*. IEEE, 373–78. doi:10.1109/IISR.2018.8535892.

5 Analyzing and Comparing MLP, CNN, and LSTM for Classification of Heart Arrhythmia Using ECG Scans

Eva Sarin, Soham Taneja, Vividha, and Preeti Nagrath
Bharati Vidyapeeth's College of Engineering

CONTENTS

INTRODUCTION

Electrocardiogram is defined as the recording of the heart's electrical activity and is often shortened as ECG. It is actually a simple and non-invasive procedure. Electrodes have to be placed on the bosom (above the abdominal region in the chest) and have to be connected in a predefined order to an apparatus and when it is switched ON, the overall activity of the heart is computed [1]. A long scroll of paper usually shows the output. The long scroll of paper is meant to describe a printed graph of the heart's activity on an electronic screen and the machine providing the output as an ECG is called an electrocardiograph. The data on the paper are further diagnosed by a medical physician. The cause of symptoms or chest pain is found with the help of an ECG. This is done by the detection of untypical heart rhythm or cardiac abnormalities, which are otherwise hard to detect. The development of Internet of things (IoT) has spawned novel ways for heart monitoring, but also presented new challenges for manual arrhythmia detection. An automated method is highly demanded to provide support for physicians. Current attempts for automatic arrhythmia detection can roughly be divided into feature-engineering-based and deep-learning-based methods. Most of the feature-engineering-based methods suffer from adopting a single classifier and they use fixed features for classifying all five types of heartbeats.

ECG has befitted as the potential primary tool in the recognition of cardiac casualties. Because of the considerably high death rate caused due to heart diseases, precise discrimination of ECG signals and early detection are important if the patients are to be cured precisely and on time. It is advised by physicians across the world to determine risks due to various factors like family heredity, diabetes, smoking, and so on [2]. Hence, ECG classification has become very important because sometimes heartbeat signals are more inclined to errors. This issue calls for a machine learning (ML) solution for analyzing the ECG data correctly. Methods of ML used for the cause of ECG processing consist of mainly three steps: signal pre-processing, noise removal methods [3], and heartbeat segmentation [4].

Feature extraction and learning/classification. Classification and detection are meant to be helpful in the identification of any deviant of the ECG signal report. Post identification of an abnormality in a patient is now replaced by an improved prognosis in the early stages of the cardiac disease or abnormality [5]. Discussion with the doctor can then provide right therapy for the patient. However, classification on ECG involves a lot of issues like deep and shallow ML methods do not show good performance when applied on asymmetrical datasets [6]. A low positive predictive value and sensitivity are acquired by most of them in respect to those classes, which have a lower sample size present in the dataset. Developing an accurate classifier that is proficient in the classification of ECG in real time has been an issue out of many [1]. Extraction and selection processes of features have been the basis of ML paradigms, which are highly dependent on the way features are designed. A surrogate procedure is to make most out of all attained information as well as allowing the ML algorithm for learning and training with the same features [7]. This is the argument backing deep learning, particularly convolutional neural networks (CNNs) and 1D-CNNs (one-dimensional convolutional neural networks), which were newly introduced for heartbeat classification specific to each patient [8], perception of myocardial infection [9], arrhythmia classification [10], detection of ectopic beats [11], and approach of sensing of arrhythmia [10] including atrial fibrillation [12] and VF [13]. Arrhythmia classification based on ECG using CNNs has had more accurate results than clinicians [14,15]. Additionally, 1D-CNNs have surpassed conventional feature extraction and feature classification paradigms for ECG beat classification [16]. If the presence of any variable segment lengths or any time dominion is detected, recurrent neural networks (RNNs) have proven to be a structured deep learning technique [17], particularly one of the alternatives like LSTM (long short term memory) networks [18,19]. LSTMs have been not only demonstrated error-free in ailments [20] but also demonstrated for detecting peculiar contractions of the heartbeat by using ECG [21,22].

Taking inspiration from the issues mentioned in the previous research works, in this chapter,

- Comparison of deep learning techniques MLP, LSTM, and CNN for classification [23] of heart arrhythmia has been proposed to be developed.
- Better summarization of their accuracies is provided by using both validation data and testing data tables each for neural network (NN), 1D-CNN, and LSTM.
- Further accuracy plots and loss plots have been obtained for trained models of NN and CNN each.
- ROC-AUC curves plotted were vital to understanding the performance of medical database models and generating a confusion matrix for the NN model on datasets consisting of the most misclassifications.

This chapter is organized as follows: Section II outlays the related work literature review in the field of DL and ECG. Section III describes the methodology including dataset description, heartbeat distinction, and model architecture. Section IV covers results and analysis, and Section V concludes the chapter.

LITERATURE REVIEW

Many researchers and clinicians have been working on ECG signal classification. They have been applying various pre-processing techniques, multiple feature extraction approaches, and classifiers. Most of them worked on the MIT-BIH arrhythmia database for the purpose of classification of ECG. ECG arrhythmia detection tasks have already seen much successful application of the conventional pattern recognition techniques, but a survey from back 2015 using not-so-conventional ML techniques shows analysis on beat selection as input and classifier's output, which is believed to be through. The survey incorporates how many beats are taken from just one file, how many classes are taken, beat selection, beat segments for classes as well as classification. Different issues in ECG classification, various noise removal preprocessing techniques, databases available for ECG, multiple classifiers based on artificial neural networks, which are available, and performance measures for determining their accuracy have been shown through an elaborated paper. The conclusion made out of this paper is that there are two ways in which ECG classification can be done, i.e., ECG signal classification and beat classification. They even called for a very less number of analysts who have explored the field of signal classification for it being a more strenuous task in comparison to beat classification. Beat classification is more difficult because normal signals of ECG can vary with every patient as at times some disease shows different signs on two different signals of ECG and it is possible that two diseases, which are completely different, show more or less similar effects on signals of ECG. Techniques or approaches mostly used for the case of preprocessing and feature extraction are algorithms like the Pan–Tompkins algorithm. In particular, the MIT-BIH arrhythmia database used for the cause of beat classification and classifier is taken as a NN have led to the observation that MLPNN (multilayer perceptron neural network) shows better accuracy for ECG beat classification has been concluded by the paper.

The deep learning-based frameworks, which had been formerly trained on a general image dataset, have shown in recent studies that frameworks were transferred in order to execute ECG arrhythmia diagnostics, supposedly automatic, through the classification of ECG of a patient. AlexNet, which is a transferred deep CNN, is being executed as a feature extractor. For the process of final classification, features that had been extracted have to be suckled into a simple backpropagation NN [5,6]. As soon as the evaluation of all the tested networks was done, the training phase showed a recognition rate and an accuracy of about 100% and above 96%, respectively. This was evaluated by transferred DL feature extraction (N-Fc6 and N-Fc7)-based networks, which was quite high as compared to the accuracies deduced from the network not based on a deep learning framework, i.e., around 90%. Some studies used deep learning architectures in which feature extractors are the first layers of convolutional neurons and some FCN layers are responsible for finally determining ECG classes with a special focus on DL using FCN (fully convolutional network) layers in the end [23,24]. The presumption made is that the absence of any medical or related subject specialists and the ability of an algorithm to extract features are highly useful for feature engineering. But the noteworthy drawbacks highlighted by authors during the implementation of algorithms are aggrieved when other deep learning solutions are compared with reference to optimization methods, proposed architecture, and computational complexity with the main open problem diagnosed as not being able to figure out the exact type of architecture to be implemented [25,26].

Taking account of the proposed structure with no straightforward feature selection technique, a ten-fold stratified cross-validation showed an overall F-measure of

0.83.10 ± 0.015 on the held-out test data (mean ± standard deviation over all folds) and 0.80 on the hidden dataset of the challenge entry server with the insistence on CNNs and RNNs especially LSTM [27,28] that focuses on refining the deep learning-based automatic framework for minimizing the issues of overestimation, information loss, and overcoming class imbalance problem as well.

In some studies [28,29], the authors ought to develop a DL network-based system that is automated and non-invasive to perform the task of basic ECG data classification whether it belongs to normal or abnormal ECG by applying DL algorithms like recurrent structures such as RNNs, long short term memory (LSTM), CNN, and gated recurrent unit (GRU). They further compared the performance using each of these architectures and obtained an accuracy of 0.834. The zenith of their method proposed approach is that there is no requirement of noise filtering or any mechanisms related to feature engineering. The results acquired prove it better than the previously published works in the basic classification of ECG. At the same point in time, the authors emphasized that although appreciative results have been encountered through DL techniques, there is not sufficient understanding of deep learning-based networks regarding their complex inner mechanisms that still remain an issue. Another similar study lodged a robust framework featuring DNNs (deep learning NNs) for automated arrhythmia classification with DNNs, bidirectional LSTM layers, and RNNs [29,30]. This work has used the CPSC database, which basically validates the performance of their framework that shows a high overall $F1$ score of 0 when present among various noises in 12 leads ECG recordings [31]. The results for this classification also show significantly increased accuracy for classification of different arrhythmias with DNNs. To add to this, their approach also illustrated improved performance with low classification error, automatic feature extraction, and anti-noise interference.

LSTMs have also proved quite influential on solutions to overcome drawbacks set by complex DL algorithms when [6,7] worked on a mixed CNN and LSTM deep learning architectural framework to detect lethal ventricular arrhythmia [32]. The results have shown that their framework outplays conventional ML algorithms. It also shows that only CNN layers-based deep learning architectures have been suggested to date for the same task. Moreover, to figure out this model, conditions are suitable in the low-end hardware of an automated external defibrillator (AED), but carrying it out on an AED is economically efficient due to its requirement of only change in software to the device. Meanwhile some authors proposed in their studies [27,34,] an LSTM network paired with focal loss (FL) improvement in training effect by curbing influence on model training caused due to the heavy number of easy normal ECG beat data. In their model, LSTM has been paired with a recurrence network model with FL, Deep learning, 1D CNN, and SVM. The results showed an accuracy of 99.26%, a recall of 99.26%, a precision of 99.30%, a specificity of 99.14%, and an $F1$ score of 99.27%. The results by experiments on their database express the effectiveness of their LSTM with FL. This method has been of great use in telemedicine scenarios for assisting cardiologists toward a more precise and objective diagnosis of ECG data signals (Table 5.1).

TABLE 5.1
Comparison of Previous Approaches

S. No.	Title	Approach	Results
1	Cardiac arrhythmia detection using deep learning [6]	Deep learning and convolutional neural networks	The testing phase obtained 98.51% and 97.53% testing recognition and average accuracy of 92.4% and 91.2% for N-Fc7 and N-Fc6 respectively
2	Deep learning for ECG analysis [24]	Deep learning and FCN Layers	Best accuracy on validation data of about 86%
3	A sequence-to-sequence deep learning approach in inter and intrapatient ECG heartbeat classification for arrhythmia detection [9]	ML-based algorithms like SVM, MLP, synthetic minority over-sampling technique (SMOTE), decision trees, and reservoir computing with linear regression	Accuracy of 99.92% and 99.53% when compared with state-of-art algorithms on randomly selected dataset vs. DS2 dataset of MIT-BIH database respectively
4	Survey on the classification of ECG signals using ML techniques [2]	Wavelet transformations like DWT, CWT, and DCT, discrete Fourier transform (DFT), Stransform (ST), principal component analysis (PCA), Pan–Tompkins algorithm, Independent component analysis (ICA), and so on. Type 2 fuzzy neural networks (T2FCNN), quantum neural network (QNN), radial basis neural network (RBFNN)	SURVEY
5	Deep learning in cardiology [33]	Deep neural networks (DNNs), graphical processing units (GPUs), decision trees, support vector machines (SVMs), convolutional neural networks (CNNs), fully connected networks (FNNs) and LSTM	LV localization using CNN and the pyramid of scales (YUDB) bears an accuracy of 98.66%

(Continued)

TABLE 5.1 (*CONTINUED*)
Comparison of Previous Approaches

S. No.	Title	Approach	Results
6	Detection of arrhythmia using an effective LSTM recurrent neural network on an imbalanced ECG dataset [27]	LSTM, FL, deep learning, 1D CNN, and SVM	LSTM network with FL ($\gamma = 2$) results in 99.26% accuracy
7	Detection of cardiac arrhythmia from ECG using a combination of convolutional and LSTM networks [28]	CNNs, RNNs, and LSTM	Best $F1$ of 83.30% with $\sigma = 1.80$
8	Using deep learning techniques, automated detection of cardiac arrhythmia from ECG [29]	Deep learning, CNN, RNN, LSTM, and GRU	Five-fold cross-validation accuracy of 0.837 after CNN 3 layer with GRU
9	Automated classification of cardiac arrhythmia using a combination of deep residual network and bidirectional LSTM [30]	DNNs, bidirectional LSTM layers, recurrent neural network (RNN)	A high overall $F1$ score of 0.806 in the presence of the different noises in the 12 leads ECG recordings on the CPSC database
10	Detection of lethal ventricular arrhythmia using mixed convolutional and LSTM [7]	1D-CNN layers, LSTM network	BAC above 99% in a public database and above 97% for the OHCA database

METHODOLOGY

DESCRIPTION OF A DATASET

The MIT-BIH arrhythmia database has been chosen. The dataset includes 48 half-hour excerpts of two-channel ambulatory ECG recordings. The recordings were obtained from 47 individuals studied by the BIH Arrhythmia Laboratory between 1975 and 1979. Twenty-three recordings were chosen randomly from a set of 4,000 24-hour ambulatory ECG recordings, which were accumulated from a diverse community of outpatients (~40%) and inpatients (~60%) at Boston's Beth Israel Hospital. The same set was the contributor to the rest of the 25 recordings as well to include not-so-common but clinically potential arrhythmias that were hardly well represented in a small random sample dataset [34]. The patients consisted of both women and men within the age of 23–89 and 32–89 years respectively. The number of each considered was 22 women and 25 men (Figures 5.1–5.4).

The recordings have been digitized at 360 samples per second per channel with 11-bit resolution over a 10 mV range. Every record was elucidated by two or more cardiologists independently. Disagreements were set on for obtaining approximately 110,000 reference annotations that can be easily read by a computer for every beat present on the dataset.

The heart possesses a conduction system separate from any other system. The PQRST complex is made up of the conduction system that we see on paper.

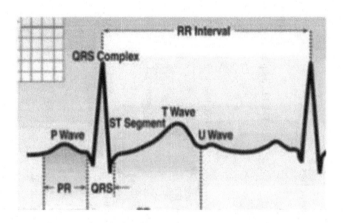

FIGURE 5.1   Conduction system [35].

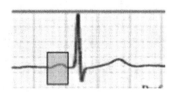

FIGURE 5.2   SA node [35].

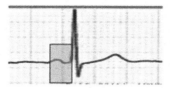

FIGURE 5.3   AV node [36].

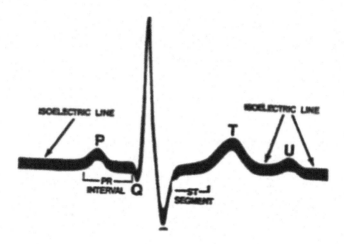

FIGURE 5.4   EKG trace.

An arrhythmia is a disruption of the conduction system [34]. For understanding and identifying arrhythmias, it is important to understand how the heart conducts normally. Arrhythmia is defined as an issue with the rate or rhythm of one's heartbeat, which refers to that the heart beats either too quickly or too slowly or in an irregular pattern.

In the case of a heart beating faster than normal, the condition is termed tachycardia. On the other hand, in the case of the heart beating too slow, the condition is termed bradycardia. Nevertheless, atrial fibrillation remains the most common type of arrhythmia [25]. It causes an irregular and fast heartbeat. However, there are many factors that can affect the rhythm of the heart, like during a heart attack, congenital heart defects, smoking, as well as stress. Drugs or medicines can also be a cause of arrhythmias.

Data Augmentation

The ECG images of the heart are studied as below (Figure 5.5):

The normal sinus rhythm in which the sinus node is the primary pacemaker, (i) one upright uniform p-wave for every QRS, (ii) the rhythm is regular, and (iii) rate= 60–100 beats/minute [6] (Figure 5.6).

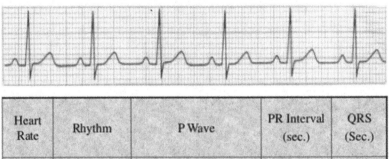

Heart Rate	Rhythm	P Wave	PR Interval (sec.)	QRS (Sec.)
60 - 100	Regular	Before each QRS, Identical	.12 - .20	<.12

FIGURE 5.5   Normal sinus rhythm [35].

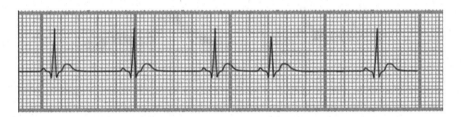

FIGURE 5.6   Supraventricular premature heart [35].

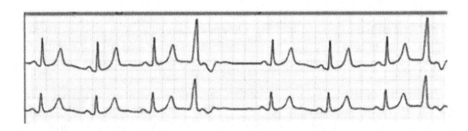

FIGURE 5.7   Premature ventricular contraction [35].

A supraventricular premature heart is that which originates in the atria. (i) One ectopic P wave and no QRS complex, (ii) rhythm is irregular, and (iii) the rate is not applicable with the PR interval (s) of 0.12–0.20 and QRS (s) of less than 0.12 [6] (Figure 5.7).

Premature ventricular contraction, (i) no p waves associated with pre-mature beat, (ii) the rhythm is irregular, and (iii) the rate is variable with PR interval (s) not known and QRS (s) wide and greater than 0.12 [6] (Figure 5.8).

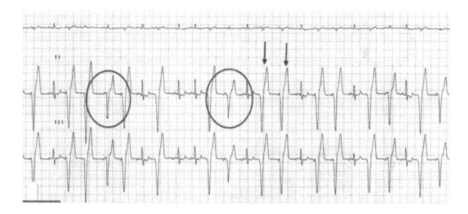

FIGURE 5.8 Fusion of ventricular and normal beats [36].

The results of the fusion of ventricular and normal beats is (i) no p waves associated to QRS, (ii) the rhythm is regular, and (iii) the rate is 100–250 beats per minute with PR interval (s) not known and QRS (s) greater than 0.12 [6].

INTERNET OF THINGS (IoT) APPROACH

IoT-based systems can monitor the heartbeat from an output given by a hardware system consisting of a NodeMCU and pulse-sensor based on Arduino. The system is based on a portable heart rate monitoring system designed in a cost-efficient manner. The prototype can also store the data of the heartbeat as well as other details of the patient and this can be used by the doctor to analyze the heart condition of the patient and for other future purposes. Early recognition of the disease is very vital in preventing more complications in the future.

The prototype blinks LED on pin 13 of the Arduino board to a user's live heartbeat, whereas "Fancy Fade Blink" on LED on pin 5 to a user's live heartbeat is signified. Here is where the users' beat-per-minute (BPM) is calculated. After the completion of this protocol, the user's IBI, which is the inter-beat interval (meaning time interval between two heartbeats), is calculated. Both the calculations of IBI and BPM use Arduino's timer interrupt. Outputs signals are obtained with BPM and IBI to serial, so that output can be used right away with the Arduino Serial Plotter.

NodeMCU is an open-source IoT platform. It is based on ESP8266 WI-FI Soc from Espressif systems. The hardware is based on an ESP-12 module. It uses the Lua scripting language. NodeMCU uses an on-module flash-based SPIFFS file system. A pulse sensor or heart rate sensor is a plug-and-play type sensor. The normal operating voltage is +5 V or +3.3 V and the current consumption is 4 mA. The sensor shown in Figure 5.9 has two sides, one side consists of an LED with an ambient light sensor and the other side contains circuitry, which amplifies the signals and filters the noise.

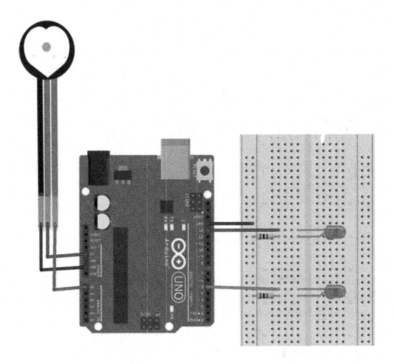

FIGURE 5.9 Arduino-based BPM [37].

FEATURE SELECTION VIA NEURAL NETWORKS

A set of those ML techniques were primarily designed for the brain with no aim to simulate it. NNs are function approximation methods with input x taken as generic signal, text, sound, or image (or any two paired up) and the output y belongs to the same set as of x, but the content present in it is more informative [33]. The formula to show the goal of NNs' intents to determine parameters for θ:

$$f\left(x{:}\theta\right) = \hat{y} \tag{5.1}$$

where

    f = predefined function
    $\hat{y}$ = prediction obtained.

But θ has certain constraints such as it should show the least possible value of cost function $J(\theta)$.

The foundation units of NNs had been laid down for the first time in 1958 [38]. It shows x as it inputs (or its summation), whereas the strength of connections is w (or its summation) and b is determined successively by x and y.

The formula used for NNs is as follows:

$$z = w(T) \cdot x + b \tag{5.2}$$

w = weights, b = biases, and T = transpose.

NNs use cost functions, which are decided according to the task to be done. The true and predicted probability distributions are differentiated by cross-entropy, which also happens to depend on the method of classification [33].

FEATURE SELECTION VIA A CONVOLUTIONAL NEURAL NETWORK

A CNN is a distinct kind of MLP [1]. CNNs can be defined as those multi-layer supervised networks, which can learn features automatically from datasets (Figure 5.2]. A CNN is augmented upon three main layers. Since years of research and implementation, CNNs have attained state-of-the-art performance with most of the essential tasks of classification [39]. The primary disadvantage that has been encountered is that they need a quite heavy and big dataset to be trained upon. However, it has been illustrated from recent studies that state-of-the-art performance is achievable with networks, which are trained on "generic" data, hence increasing the likelihood for the development of a place recognition system established based on the features acquired from datasets focused on classification [39]. Spatial sampling, weight sharing, and local connection are crucial traits of a CNN [21]. It provides most of the feature data for not only training the model but also classification. However, it requires a considerable quantity of computation as well. A CNN's structure consists of three convolution layers, two max pool layers, and one fully connected layer.

The equation to be taken during the training is as follows:

$$Z = X * F \tag{5.3}$$

where
X = input, F = filter, and $*$ = convolution operation.

The convolutional layer's output is forwarded to the pooling layer. It consists of a ReLU function activation, which uses a max $(0, X)$ to every input X of the ReLU function. The max-pooling operation pertained to every feature map derives the most important features, which means selecting features with the highest values. Now the features, which have been selected, are fed to the fully connected layer, possessing a function called softmax, which provides probability distribution over each class. Therefore, the final output class is computed by the fully connected layer (FC), which was obtained from the CNN [7].

FEATURE SELECTION VIA LSTM

LSTM is defined as a time-recurrent NN. LSTM is believed to work for time-series prediction of crucial events. Its delay interval is relatively long [38]. A NN is suitable for effectively retaining historical information further realizing the learning of long-term dependence information of text [27]. Basically, LSTM has an input gate, forget gate, output gate, and a cell unit so that it can update and retain the historical information (Figure 5.3).

The forget gate $F(t)$ in the LSTM memory block is handled by only one neuron. It decides which information should be retained and which should be discarded to allow the storage of historical information. The input gate $U(t)$ is where the LSTM block is created by a neuron and the previous memory unit is affected. The reason behind its activation is to determine whether the historical information should be updated. The selected update content out of the information $C'(t)$ is calculated by $\tan h$. The current time memory cell is then calculated by the current candidate cell, the previous time state, and the input gate information $U(t)$, and the forget gate information $F(t)*O(t)$ of the LSTM block at the current time is produced at the output gate. Finally, $a(t)$ finds the quantity of information regarding the current cell state that should be the output. The following are the steps and activations used:

$$F(t) = \text{sigmoid}\left(Wf\left[a(t-1),\ x(t)\right] + bf\right) \tag{5.4}$$

$$U(t) = \text{sigmoid}\left(Wu\left[a(t-1),\ x(t)\right] + bu\right) \tag{5.5}$$

$$C'(t) = \tan h\left(Wc\left[a(t-1),\ x(t)\right] + bc\right) \tag{5.6}$$

$$O(t) = \text{sigmoid}\left(Wo\left[a(t-1),\ x(t)\right] + bo\right) \tag{5.7}$$

$$C(t) = U(t)*C'(t) + F(t)*C(t-1) \tag{5.8}$$

$$a(t) = O(t)\tan\tan h\left(C(t)\right)$$

Activations used in the above mentioned equations:

$$\text{sigmoid}(x) = \frac{1}{1+e^{-x}} \tag{5.9}$$

$$\text{relu}(x) = \max(0,x) \tag{5.10}$$

$$\text{softmax}(x) = \frac{e^x}{\text{sum}\left(e^{Xi}\right)}$$

After determining the hidden vector for every position, the last hidden vector was taken into consideration as the ECG signal representation. The LSTM was fed to a linear layer along with an output length of the classification number. It was then added to a softmax output layer to classify the ECG beat [27].

In this chapter, a five-layer LSTM architecture including an input layer has been setup. It has been shown in Figure 5.3.

ALGORITHM PROPOSED (FIGURES 5.10–5.12)

1. Input 180 data points from ECG sensor.
   Upsample the minority classes using SMOTE.
   Store these data points into an array.
   Store the one hot encoded labels to another array.
   Model Creation:
   5a. Fully Connected:

```
fc_model = Sequential()
fc_model.add(Dense(64,activation = 'relu', input_shape = (187,)))
fc_model.add(Dropout(.2))
fc_model.add(Dense(128,activation = 'relu'))
fc_model.add(Dropout(.2))
fc_model.add(Dense(256,activation = 'relu'))
fc_model.add(Dropout(.2))
fc_model.add(Dense(128,activation = 'relu'))
fc_model.add(Dropout(.2))
fc_model.add(Dense(5,activation = 'softmax'))
```

```
fc_model.compile(optimizer = keras.optimizers.Nadam(0.0001), loss = 'categorical_crossentropy', metrics = ['accuracy'])
```

```
lr = ReduceLROnPlateau(factor = 0.5,patience = 2)
mc = ModelCheckpoint('fc_model1.h5', save_best_only=True)
fc_hist = fc_model.fit(train_x_up, train_y_up, validation_data = (test_x, test_y), epochs = 15,batch_size = 64,callbacks = [lr, mc], initial_epoch=0)
fc_model.evaluate(val_x, val_y)
```

5b. CNN:

```
cnn_model = Sequential()
cnn_model.add(Conv1D(128,(3), activation = 'relu', input_shape = (187,1), padding = 'same'))
cnn_model.add(BatchNormalization())
cnn_model.add(MaxPool1D((3), (2), padding = 'same'))
cnn_model.add(Conv1D(64,(3), activation = 'relu', padding = 'same'))
cnn_model.add(BatchNormalization())
cnn_model.add(MaxPool1D((3), (2), padding = 'same'))
cnn_model.add(Conv1D(64,(3), activation = 'relu', padding = 'same'))
cnn_model.add(BatchNormalization())
cnn_model.add(MaxPool1D((3), (2), padding = 'same'))
cnn_model.add(Flatten())
cnn_model.add(Dense(128,activation = 'relu'))
cnn_model.add(Dense(64,activation = 'relu'))
cnn_model.add(Dense(5,activation = 'softmax'))
```

```
cnn_model.compile(optimizer = 'adam',          loss = 'categorical_crossentropy', metrics = ['accuracy'])
```

```
cnn_hist = cnn_model.fit(train_x2,train_y_up, validation_data = (test_x2,test_y),
epochs = 15,batch_size = 64,callbacks = [lr, mc])
```
5c LSTM:
```
lstm_model = Sequential()
lstm_model.add(keras.layers.Bidirectional(keras.layers.
LSTM(64,input_shape = (187,1))))
lstm_model.add(Dropout(0.2))
lstm_model.add(Dense(5,activation='softmax'))

lstm_model.compile(optimizer = 'adam',        loss = 'categorical_crossentropy',
metrics = ['accuracy'])

lstm_model.fit(train_x2,train_y_up, validation_data = (test_x2,test_y), epochs = 5,
batch_size = 1024,callbacks = [lr, mc])
```
6. Analyze the model performance on the test set.

MODEL ARCHITECTURE (FIGURE 5.13)

EXPERIMENTAL SETUP

The experimental setup used in this project utilizes the google colab's docker virtual environment consisting of Nvidia P100 GPU with 16 GB vRAM, Intel Xeon Processor, and 13 GB of RAM. Apart from this, 64GB of disk space was available. The given data are cleaned and normalized. The dataset is split in a ratio of 80:20 for training and validation. For the predictions, three models, NN, CNN, and LSTM, are chosen. All three models are trained to predict the five labels. Performance is measured by calculating precision and recall metrics.

RESULTS AND ANALYSIS

NEURAL NETWORK

Validation Data:
    Testing Data:

1D CONVOLUTIONAL NEURAL NETWORK

Validation Data:
    Testing Data:

LSTM

Validation Data:
    Testing Data:
    These metrics are evaluated over five labels in the dataset explained as follows:
    N for the normal beat, S for the supraventricular premature beat, V for the premature ventricular contraction, F for the fusion of ventricular and normal beats, and Q for the unclassifiable beat NN on testing data.

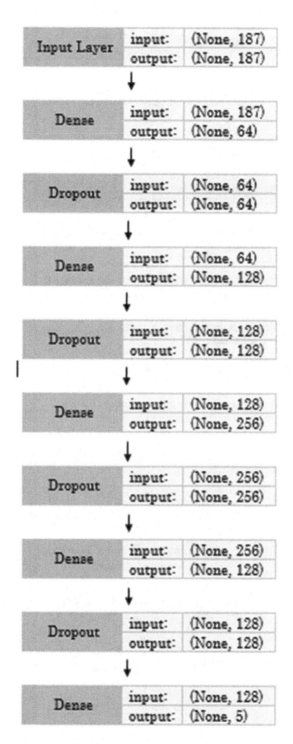

FIGURE 5.10 Architecture of layers in a NN.

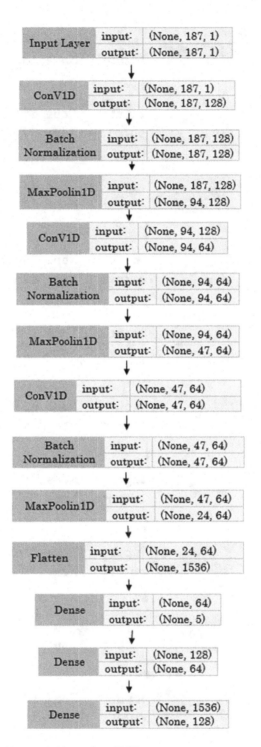

FIGURE 5.11   Architecture of layers in a CNN.

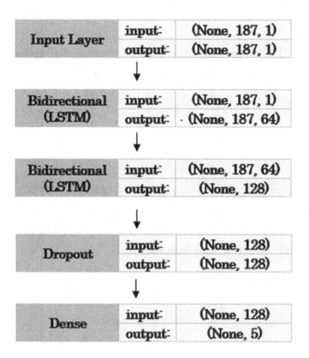

FIGURE 5.12 Architecture of layers in an LSTM.

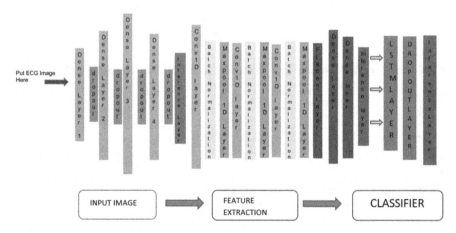

FIGURE 5.13 Model proposed architecture.

Tables 5.2, 5.4, and 5.6 represent the classification report of the model on the validation dataset. It can be seen clearly that on validation data, both the CNN and LSTM models perform equally well.

Tables 5.3, 5.5, and 5.7 represent the classification report of the model on the testing dataset. Although the LSTM model performs well on the validation dataset, but on newer data, the CNN network supersedes the other models.

TABLE 5.2

Precision, Recall, *F*1-score, and Accuracy in a NN on Validation Data

Label	Precision	Recall	*F*1-Score
N	0.99	0.97	0.98
S	0.53	0.81	0.64
V	0.9	0.93	0.91
F	0.61	0.84	0.71
Q	0.97	0.98	0.97
Accuracy			0.96

TABLE 5.3

Precision, Recall, *F*1-score, and Accuracy

Label	Precision	Recall	*F*1-Score
N	0.93	0.97	0.95
S	0.84	0.76	0.8
V	0.96	0.93	0.94
F	0.77	0.83	0.8
Q	0.99	0.97	0.98
Accuracy			0.94

TABLE 5.4

Precision, Recall, *F*1-score, and Accuracy in a CNN on Validation Data

Label	Precision	Recall	*F*1-Score
N	0.99	1	0.99
S	0.9	0.82	0.86
V	0.97	0.96	0.96
F	0.82	0.81	0.81
Q	1	0.99	0.99
Accuracy			0.99

TABLE 5.5

Precision, Recall, *F*1-Score, and Accuracy in a CNN on Testing Data

Label	Precision	Recall	*F*1-Score
N	0.94	0.99	0.97
S	0.97	0.79	0.87
V	0.99	0.95	0.97
F	0.83	0.86	0.85

TABLE 5.6
Precision, Recall, *F*1-Score, and Accuracy in an LSTM on Validation Data

Label	Precision	Recall	*F*1-Score
N	0.99	1	0.99
S	0.9	0.82	0.86
V	0.97	0.96	0.96
F	0.82	0.81	0.81
Q	1	0.99	0.99
Accuracy			0.99

TABLE 5.7
Precision, Recall, *F*1-Score, and Accuracy in an LSTM on Testing Data

Label	Precision	Recall	*F*1-Score
N	0.98	0.95	0.97
S	0.61	0.72	0.66
V	0.85	0.89	0.87
F	0.3	0.87	0.44
Q	0.9	0.94	0.92
Accuracy			0.94

ACCURACY AND LOSS PLOTS

The plots below are used to monitor the model-training performance.

Learning parameters influence the results of experiments carried out and their impact has been computably analyzed to obtain the best learning parameters for our model. Evaluation of classification accuracy of the results via experiment of more than one case on the testing set helped us in the derivation of the optimal parameter value [27].

The accuracy plots indicate that the model performance improves and raises with the number of epochs and loss reduces, which is desirable.

NN

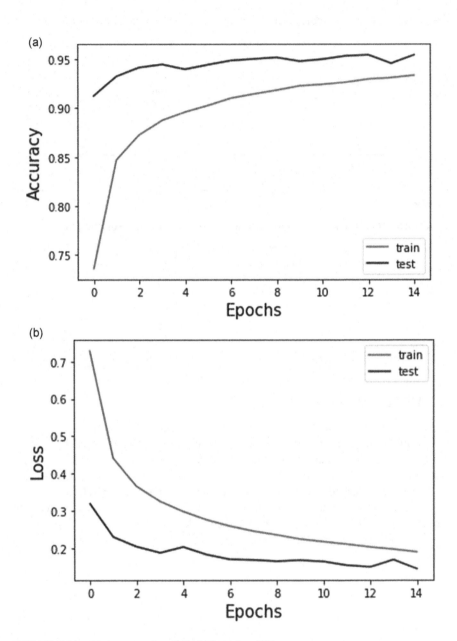

FIGURE 5.14   (a) Accuracy in a NN, (b) Loss in a NN.

CNN

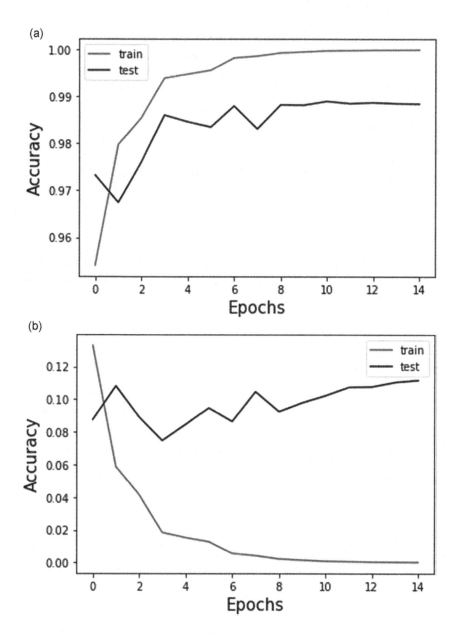

FIGURE 5.15   (a) Accuracy in a CNN, (b) Loss in a CNN.

Figure 5.14a and 5.15a represent the training accuracy of the NN and LSTM model respectively, for 15 epochs. Accuracies can be clearly seen increasing with the successive epochs, hence concluding that our models are training as expected.

Figures 5.14b and 5.15b represent the training loss of the NN and LSTM model respectively, for 15 epochs. The loss of the CNN model is lower and decays as desired. Hence, both the models achieve low losses after the training is complete.

Note – The plots for LSTM models are not shown since the LSTM models take a longer time to train and hence, they have only been trained for two epochs.

ROC-AUC CURVES

NN

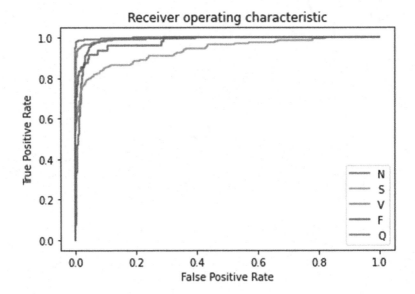

FIGURE 5.16 TP rate vs. FP rate in a NN.

CNN

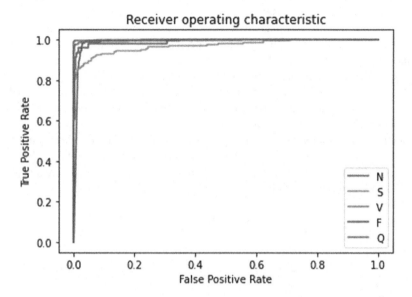

FIGURE 5.17   TP rate vs. FP rate in a CNN.

LSTM

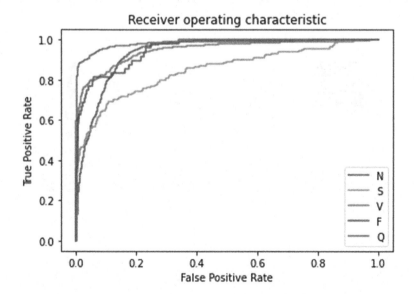

FIGURE 5.18   TP rate vs. FP rate in an LSTM.

Figures 5.16–5.18 represent the receiver operating characteristic curves for NN, CNN, and LSTM models respectively. These curves are vital to understand the performance of medical data-based models.

We can see that the relationship between the false-positive rate and the true-positive rate is preserved. Also, the graph has been concentrated around the left corner on the top (TPR ~ 1.0, FPR ~ 0.0).

Figure 5.19 presents the confusion matrix. This confusion matrix is for the NN model on the test set. It represents the classified labels against the original labels. It can be observed that most of the data is concentrated in class 0 (normal ECG) and hence consists of the most misclassifications.

Accuracy, specificity, and sensitivity of the classification are the three main measurement performances on NN models on whose ground the performance has been appraised. A confusion matrix has been used to describe these measurements [40].

These are explained as follows:

Precision is calculated as the ratio of true positives (TP) to the sum of TP and
    false positives (FP)
Precision = TP/(TP+FP)
The recall is calculated as the ratio of TP to the sum of TP and false negatives
    (FN)
Recall = TP/(TP+FN)

A confusion matrix is defined as a matrix (table) that is used to determine the performance of an ML algorithm under supervised learning preferably. The row of a confusion matrix expresses instances of a real class and the column is meant to express instances of a predicted class [39].

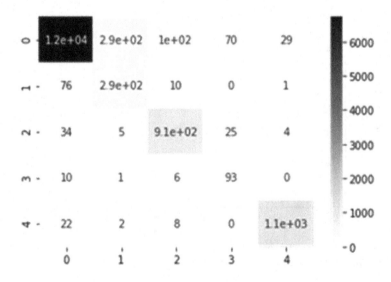

FIGURE 5.19   Confusion matrix for a NN on test data.

As shown, the proposed model had made mistakes where the top right and bottom left outputs of the matrix are understandably wrong while the top left and bottom left values of the matrix are correct predictions of the NN model [41].

CONCLUSIONS AND FUTURE WORK

The proposed chapter represents a novel and effective ECG classification using one-dimensional CNN alongside FCN layers using IoT-based PBM on preprocessed time-series data. The accuracy of the results as achieved from the validation data via the accuracy charts is quite high and the losses assessed are quite low as well in the CNN model. The classifier model is built with different kinds of feature sets. The proposed IoT-enabled PBM with statistical and dynamic features has significant potential in improving the accuracy of the classifier. Although the drawbacks that surfaced were over-fitting due to limited resources of the dataset, the database that has been used is the MIT-BIH arrhythmia database and the results on it prove the robustness of the setup.

Future work will focus on:

1. Gathering more training data and increasing the classified beats.
2. Using more robust models, such as BiLSTM, and reducing over-fitting.
3. Relaying data from the sensor to evaluate real-time performance.
4. Cleaning outliers and evaluating performance on new data.
5. Increasing the accuracy to be obtained from the LSTM-based model due to low availability of epochs. Due to the same, the time processed was as 10× as compared to CNN and NN.

REFERENCES

1. Mousavi S, Fatemeh Afghah School of Informatics, Computing and Cyber Systems, Northern Arizona University, USA 'Inter-and intra-patient ECG heartbeat classification for arrhythmia detection: a sequence to sequence deep learning approach', *IEEE International Conference on Acoustics, Speech and Signal Processing (ICASSP)*, Brighton, United Kingdom, 2019, pp. 1308–1312, doi: 10.1109/ICASSP.2019.8683140.
2. Jambukia SH, Dabhi VK, Prajapati HB, Classification of ECG signals using machine learning techniques: a survey, *International Conference on Advances in Computer Engineering and Applications (ICACEA)*, IMS Engineering College, Ghaziabad, India, 2015, doi: 10.1109/ICACEA.2015.7164783.
3. Moody GB, Mark RG. The impact of the MIT-BIH arrhythmia database. *IEEE Engineering in Medicine and Biology*. 2001; 20(3):45–50. PMID: 11446209.
4. Goldberger AL, Amaral LAN, Glass L, Hausdorff JM, Ivanov PCh, Mark RG, Mietus JE, Moody GB, Peng C-K, Stanley HE. Components of new research resources for physiologic signals PhysioBank, Physio Toolkit. *Circulation*. 2000; 101:e215–e220. doi: 10.1161/01.CIR.101.23.e215.
5. Isina A, Ozdalili S, Cardiac arrhythmia detection using deep learning, *9th International Conference on Theory and Application of Soft Computing, Computing with Words and Perception, ICSCCW 2017*, 24–25 August 2017, Budapest, Hungary, ISBN: 978-1-5108-5591-5.
6. Picon A, Irusta U, lvarez Gila AA, Aramend E, Alonso-Atienza F, Figuera C, Ayala U, Garrote E, Wik L, Kramer-Johansen J, Eftestøl T, Mixed convolutional and long short-term memory network for the detection of lethal ventricular arrhythmia. *PLoS One*. 2019; 14(5):e0216756.

7. Kiranyaz S, Ince T, Gabbouj M, Real-time patient-specific ECG classification by 1-D convolutional neural networks. *IEEE Transactions on Biomedical Engineering.* 2016; 63(3):664–675. doi: 10.1109/TBME.2015.2468589, PMID: 26285054.

8. Acharya UR, Fujita H, Lih OS, Hagiwara Y, Tan JH, Adam M, Automated detection of arrhythmias using different intervals of tachycardia ECG segments with convolutional neural network. *Information Sciences.* 2017; 405:81–90. doi: 10.1016/j.ins.2017.04.012.

9. Acharya UR, Fujita H, Lih OS, Hagiwara Y, Tan JH, Adam M, Application of deep convolutional neural network for automated detection of myocardial infarction using ECG signals. *Information Sciences.* 2017; 405. doi: 10.1016/j.ins.2017.04.012.

10. Al Rahhal MM, Bazi Y, Al Zuair M, Othman E, BenJdira B, Convolutional neural networks for electrocardiogram classification. *Journal of Medical and Biological Engineering.* 2018; 38(6):1014–1025.

11. Xia Y, Wulan N, Wang K, Zhang H, Detecting atrial fibrillation by deep convolutional neural networks. *Computers in Biology and Medicine.* 2018; 93:84–92. doi: 10.1016/j.compbiomed.2017.12.007, PMID: 29291535.

12. Acharya UR, Fujita H, Oh SL, Raghavendra U, Tan JH, Adam M, Gertych A, Hagiwara Y, Automated identification of shockable and non-shockable life-threatening ventricular arrhythmias using convolutional neural network. *Future Generation Computers.* 2017; 79:952–959. doi: 10.1016/j.future.2017.08.039.

13. Rajpurkar P, Hannun AY, Haghpanahi M, Bourn C, Ng AY. Cardiologist-level arrhythmia detection with convolutional neural networks. *Nature Medicine.* 2017; 2019. doi: 10.1038/s41591-019-0359-9. PMID: 30679787.

14. Hannun AY, Rajpurkar P, Haghpanahi M, Tison GH, Bourn C, Turakhia MP, Ng AY, Cardiologist-level arrhythmia detection and classification in ambulatory electrocardiograms using a deep neural network. *Nature Medicine.* 2019; 25:65–69. doi: 10.1038/s41591-018-0268-3. PMID: 30617320.

15. Ince T, Zabihi M, Kiranyaz S, Gabbouj M, Learned vs. hand-designed features for ECG beat classification: a comprehensive study. In: Eskola H, Väisänen O, Viik J, Hyttinen J (eds) *EMBEC & NBC 2017.* Singapore: Springer; 2017, pp. 551–554.

16. Graves A, *Supervised Sequence Labelling with Recurrent Neural Networks.* Berlin, Heidelberg: Springer; 2012, vol. 385 of Studies in Computational Intelligence.

17. Hochreiter S, Schmidhuber J, Long short-term memory. *Neural Computation.* 1997; 9(8):1735–1780.

18. Gers FA, Schmidhuber J, Cummins F, Learning to forget: continual prediction with LSTM. Neural computation. *Proceedings of the ICANN'99 International Conference on Artificial Neural Networks* (Edinburgh, Scotland), 1999, vol. 2, pp. 850–855. IEEE, London 2000.

19. Lipton ZC, Kale DC, Elkan C, Wetzell R, Learning to diagnose with LSTM recurrent neural networks. Published as a Conference Paper at *ICLR 2016.* arXiv:1511.03677.

20. Chauhan S, Vig L., Anomaly detection in ECG time signals via deep long short-term memory networks. *2015 IEEE International Conference on Data Science and Advanced Analytics (DSAA);* 2015, pp. 1–7, Paris, France.

21. Goldberger AL, Amaral LAN, Glass L, Hausdorff JM, Ivanov PCh, Mark RG, Mietus JE, Moody GB, Peng C-K, Stanley HE, PhysioBank, PhysioToolkit, and PhysioNet: Components of a new research resource for complex physiologic signals. *Circulation* 2000; 101(23):e215–e220.

22. Kachuee M, Fazeli S, Sarrafzadeh M, ECG heartbeat classification: a deep transferable representation. *IEEE International Conference on Healthcare Informatics (ICHI)* 2018. doi: 10.1109/ICHI.2018.00092.

23. Pyakillya B, Kazeachenko N, Mikhailovsky N, Deep learning for ECG classification. *Journal of Physics.* 2017; 913:012004. doi: 10.1088/1742-6596/913/1/012004.

24. Bizopoulos P, Koutsouris D, Deep learning in cardiology. *IEEE Reviews in Biomedical Engineering.* 2019; 12:168–193. doi: 10.1109/RBME.2018.2885714.
25. Heart and Stroke Encyclopedia (American Heart Association). Internet Source. https://medlineplus.gov/arrhythmia.html.
26. Internet Source. All about heart rate (pulse). https://www.heart.org/en/health-topics/high-blood-pressure/the-facts-about-high-blood-pressure/all-about-heart-rate-pulse.
27. ECG heartbeat categorization dataset. Internet Source. https://www.kaggle.com/shayanfazeli/heartbeat.
28. PTB diagnostic ECG database. Internet Source. https://www.physionet.org/content/ptbdb/1.0.0/.
29. MIT-BIH arrhythmia database. Internet Source. https://www.physionet.org/content/mitdb/1.0.0/.
30. Gao J, Zhang H, Lu P, Wang Z, An effective LSTM recurrent network to detect arrhythmia on imbalanced ECG dataset. *Journal of Health Care Engineering.* 2019; 2019, Article ID 6320651.
31. Warriack P, Homsi MN, Cardiac arrhythmia Detection from ECG combining convolutional and long short term memory networks. *Conference of Computing in Cardiology,* Rennes, France, 2017, vol. 44. doi: 10.22489/CinC.2017.161-460.
32. Swapna G, Soman KP, Vinayakumar R, Automated detection of cardiac arrhythmia using deep learning techniques. *International Conference on Computational Intelligence and Data Science (ICCIDS).* 2018; 132:1192–1201.
33. He R, Liu Y, Wang K, Zhao N, Yuan Y, Li Q, Zhang H, Automatic cardiac arrhythmia classification using combination of deep residual network and bidirectional LSTM. *IEEE Access.* 2019; 7:102119–102135.
34. Mungra D, Agrawal A, Sharma P, Tanwar S, Obaidat MS, *PRATIT: A CNN-Based Emotion Recognition System Using Histogram Equalization and Data Augmentation.* Springer Science &Business Media, LLC, part of Springer Nature, 2019. doi: 10.1007/s11042-019-08397-0.
35. Chen Z, Lam O, Jacobson A, Milford, M, Convolutional neural network based place recognition. *Australasian Conference on Robotics and Automation (ACRA 2014) University of Melbourne.* https://arxiv.org/abs/1411.1509.
36. Hannun AY, Rajpurkar P, Haghpanahi M, Tison GH, Bourn C, Turakhia MP, Ng AY, Cardiologist-level arrhythmia detection and classification in ambulatory electrocardiograms using a deep neural network. *Nature Medicine.* 2019; 25:65–69. doi: 10.1038/s41591-018-0268-3.
37. Pandey S, Janghel R, Vani V. Patient specific machine learning models for ECG signal classification. *Procedia Computer Science.* 2020; 167:2181–2190. doi: 10.1016/j.procs.2020.03.269.
38. Carolina Sleep Society. Internet Source. https://carolinasleepsociety.org/.
39. Rosenblatt FF, The perceptron: a probabilistic model for information storage and organization in the brain. *Psychological Review.* 1958; 65(6):386–408.
40. Sak H, Senior A, Beaufays F, Long short-term memory recurrent neural network architectures for large scale acoustic modeling. *Proceedings of the Fifteenth Annual Conference of the International Speech Communication Association,* pp. 338–342, Singapore, September 2014.
41. Getting (calculating) BPM. Internet Source. https://pulsesensor.com/pages/getting-advanced.

6 AI-Powered Robotics and COVID-19: Challenges and Opportunities

Kajol Mohanty, Subiksha S., Kirthikka S.,
Sujal B. H., Sumathi Sokkanarayanan,
Panjavarnam Bose, and
Mithileysh Sathiyanarayanan
Sri Sairam Engineering College

CONTENTS

INTRODUCTION

Nations around the globe have been affected by the COVID-19 pandemic since December 2019 [1], and the medical care facilities in these nations are quickly adjusting to the exponential challenges and demands. The World Health Organization (WHO) has called for the latest technologies to help with the reaction to the flare-up across health and wellbeing areas, and artificial intelligence (AI)-powered robotics has been distinguished as one of the most encouraging ways to tackle COVID-19 [2].

The COVID-19 pandemic is solitary from multiple points of view. To start with, as far as the number of individuals infected, contagiousness, and range of clinical seriousness are concerned, COVID-19 has had a greater impact to date than previous epidemics such as pandemic influenza, Middle East respiratory syndrome (MERS), severe acute respiratory syndrome (SARS), and Ebola virus [3]. Now, the COVID-19 pandemic is happening in a period of monstrous innovative progression. AI-powered robotics can effectively support healthcare and wellbeing areas during a pandemic by tracking health conditions in real time, creating virtual visits for day-to-day operations, and providing telemedicine visits for patients.

However, these kinds of latest technologies may pose challenges associated with barriers to access, acceptability, and ethical issues. The COVID-19 pandemic is setting a stage to examine how AI-powered robotics can and ought to be utilized to address it. This chapter outlines the current opportunities and challenges with respect to AI-powered robots to battle COVID-19.

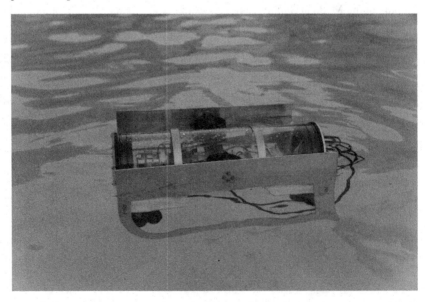

Water robots help in cleaning and sanitizing water pools. The demand for these autonomous robots is skyrocketing during this pandemic.

OPPORTUNITIES

THE GENERAL SURGE OF 3D PRINTING DURING COVID-19

The global unforeseeable caused by COVID-19 pandemic has pushed the globe into a tangled situation, which is yet to entangle. The quick product development of 3D printing accredits a prompt movement of the technology and therefore a swift response to the exigencies. The 3D printing has made it possible to manufacture critical parts on demand by leveraging designs shared via online platforms in spite of facing heavy discrepancies in the supply chain. This manifested to be really helpful in this pandemic where all the protocols of social distancing were very well managed and at the same time, the work of producing essential equipment was never put on halt. Furthermore, customization of complex designs can be availed easily due to 3D printers. The enormous demand for 3D-printing applications in tackling COVID-19 includes personal protective equipment (PPE), visualization aids, public accessories and essentials, medical and testing devices, and so on.

The introduction of 3D printing in intricate care has been fruitful. The 3D printers fabricate low-cost prosthetics for people who need them. People who are not capable of affording a prosthetic can go for the prosthetics created by 3D printers, as these are cost efficient. The 3D printing makes it easier to print the necessary equipment in those villages where regular transportation is a subject of concern.

Fitz Frames is a company that manufactures custom glasses using the latest 3D printing machines. The company has also manufactured a lot of other safety aids [4].

TESTING DONE BY AUTONOMOUS ROBOTS IN A BID TO PROTECT FRONTLINE WARRIORS

During these hard times, self-governing systems that require minimal manual operations can be of great help. Such systems can be fostered in medical centers and research labs for aiding and shielding the people working there in numerous ways and in a similar fashion, this can be beneficial to the general public. For example, robots can be used to help prevent the spread of COVID-19. The wheeled machine, which is fully remote controlled, is well versed in performing tests such as swab tests and ultrasound scans and recording the information by listening to organs with a robot stethoscope. By introducing smart telecare systems, we can turn down the risk of frontline workers getting infected by the transmission of deadly viruses by ensuring that they monitor, test, and diagnose the diseased patients from a safe distance. Diagnostic tests such as swab tests or checking a patient's temperature can be done by wheeled robots carrying manipulators to conduct such tests and this can potentially safeguard the medical staff from directly coming in contact with the diseased. Telecare systems can reduce the use of PPE for examining a patient, as it is a tough nut to crack by wearing the PPE suit and doing the treatment.

Nearly 14 robots were arranged by a Beijing-based robotics company CloudMinds to Wuhan for providing necessary help. The CloudMinds' humanoid service robot, Ginger, helped with hospital services [5].

DIGITAL COMMUNICATION DURING THE PANDEMIC

It is very crucial to keep up the communication strong between the government offi-cials and the medical authorities as well as the research team. Since the outbreak of COVID-19, there has been a lot of miscommunication and disbelief via social media, texts, SMS, and so on about the inception and transmission of the disease. Many misleading facts are present in the internet and in government disclosures regarding the same. The society and its people may be hampered by the widespread of false speculations in the public domain. The WHO is all set to provide people the correct information in a timely fashion, via an active authentic information campaign. With the betterment of communication strategies, the courage in people reinforces and thereby helps manage their fear factors and keep the risk of other health conditions such as blood pressure, heart rate, and so on under control resultantly decreasing the risk of weak immune systems. The communication must not only be comprehensible and based on true facts but also must be fast enough to reach the target community such as health workers, hospitals, and the public for them to take up immediate action wisely when necessary. Guidelines such as maintaining social distancing were mis-judged and misunderstood, as they were not well elucidated. Rather messages such as "stay home, stay safe' should have been emphasized more to avoid the spike in the number of people affected by COVID-19 daily. The WHO web page projects the usage of the phrase "physical distance" in association with "social distance." Therefore, here comes the importance of digital interaction, which helps to avoid physical contact or physical interactions and enables people to maintain social dis-tancing in person as per the WHO guidelines.

During the initial months of the pandemic, industry reports showed that there is a visible hike in the usage of digital media as people stayed home due to lockdown [6].

ROBOTIC GUIDANCE AND ASSISTANCE FOR A MUCH BETTER LIFE

Robotics is not only limited to navigating racks and tools and assisting in pathologi-cal labs, in the healthcare field. With the introduction of remote-controlled medical robots, such as the ones invented by Anybots, caretakers keep a track of the health conditions of patients, make necessary arrangements for regular check-ups, and even book appointments as per the requirement. This practice can be of great help in saving time and increasing efficiency by ruling out the doctor's visit to residents for treating patients. A company Luvozo created Sam, the robotic concierge and this was tested first in Washington DC [7]. It is a human-sized robot, it is the conglom-eration of cutting edge mechanization and human touch for assisting the medical staff in providing frequent check-ups and nursing patients personally at their resi-dents if required, and most interestingly, it has been mechanized with a machinery smiling face, which resembles a human smile to make the patients feel lively from within. This not only reduces the overhead but also at the same time, pulls up the graph of the satisfactory level of the patients high. One added advantage is that, as it is a machine, it can work continuously with better accuracy and reliability. These features make it more reliable.

ROBOTS IN THE MEDICAL SUPPLY CHAIN

Robots are known for their impeccable accuracy with a very high speed; their work ranges from moving boxes to chemical testing. We even have robots designed for testing protection clothing for the US military [8]. Robots are always prioritized in emergency situations as they are more reliable and it is always better than risking a human life in hazardous situations. Robotics medical dispenser systems, PharmASSIST robots, which have got tremendous data mining capabilities, and this practice are going to be of great help in the near future where the medical experts can save a lot of time and incentives and can invest in these resources by considering the social aspects of society such as: educating people about the preventive measures, providing practical demonstrations, and therefore making healthcare truly caring and way too effective.

PERFECT FOR DELIVERIES DURING THIS PANDEMIC

There is no rocket science to figure out that robots can be the best replacements for thousands of manual jobs. By this year, robots were presumed to be working in malls, doing commercial works and helping to deliver goods at our place. During this pandemic situation, in order to reduce the risk of infection among people, these robots will come handy. Two Skype co-founders initiated a six-wheeled robot of Starship Technologies in 2014. This special robot needed no human assistance to helm around [9].

SOCIAL ROBOTS

Healthcare medical devices are an important part of the system, which balances the insanity, stability, and comfort during quarantine so that they are socially engaging with people. It will be an inspiration and will captivate those quarantined to build up their heaps/caliber among their groups while under isolation. The main purpose of such devices' innovation is meant for senior citizens plus kids having severe illnesses. Majorly, these people have been pompous due to the pandemic because of no visitors in the health care. Undergoing such situations, these devices can be extensively used in reducing their mental sickness, regardless of being in any age group.

These medical robotic devices are developed in different types, that is, starting with pets resembling miniature till hominoids [10]. In order for making social robots more effective, various kinds of sensing elements as well as actuating elements are feasibly introduced in them [11–13].

TELEMEDICINE AND REMOTE PATIENT MONITORING SYSTEMS

In order to avoid the overcrowding of emergency rooms during COVID-19, telemedicine plays a pivotal role by allowing patients to stay and receive care at home whenever required. Telemedicine allows regular basic medical care and electronics prescriptions besides secured bracing of COVID-19 patients. It is also beneficial to professionals as they can screen and scan symptoms and provide helpful medical advice to the patients at home. This keeps patients away from overloaded hospitals.

A potential study regarding COVID-19 severity was carried out in Luxembourg (Predi-COVID). The data were extracted from the national telesurveillance system, which had utilized data of all patients that had tested positive for COVID-19. The collected information is integrated with the patient's reported results and biological illustrations. There are ingenious data collections such as the voice recording based on smartphones, which is used to recognize respiratory syndromes due to vocal biomarkers.

BENEFITS OF ROBOTIC SURGERY

Surgery using robots can be carried out in a less inhibitory manner with the surgeon handling the robot at a distance. Hence, treatment of the patients can be done with a minimal number of nurses or caretakers, which in turn reduces the expense. This also benefits the quality of healthcare for the patient. In addition, doctors might become unfocused due to weariness or fatigue. Therefore, it becomes stressful for surgeons to operate at long stretches of time, which could lead to huge blunders. On the other hand, surgery using robots could change all of this and would beat all these odds. Robotic surgery will allow much greater and better precision during neurological or orthopedic surgeries. Stryker is the second-dominant competitor in the market of robotic surgery, after the possession of MAKO Surgical Corp in 2013 for $1.65 billion.

TRIAGE AND RISK MANAGEMENT

There is an alarming situation in the world, which has created uncertainty among all of us. In order to assure the allocation of resources, video conferences can be very helpful in comforting patients and also at the time of trials. At first, patients are designated as possibly COVID-19 infected or uninfected prior to their arrival at hospitals. On top of it, telemedicine ensures keen monitoring of patients at home who are less severely infected by constant communication. The next phase usually occurred at hospitals where severely infected COVID patients are televised by a lively evaluation of immunological characteristics and testing. These patients are isolated in emergency rooms, where they are provided with android (or apple) devices to talk to professionals; these electronic gadgets are sanitized regularly. A robot enters this place to observe the vital and cardiac signs. These robots come in handy to reduce contamination among healthcare providers. They also act as an interface between patients and healthcare professionals. Their activities are controlled by nurses some-where out of that room. Symptoms check, consultations, and prescription can be done online. Basically, low-risk people can be kept track from their homes regularly. Moreover, severely infected patients can be evaluated with the help of these robots.

In order to measure temperature, breathing rate, pulse, and oxygen saturation and to make them mobile, researchers have decided to utilize prevailing computer vision technologies.

CHALLENGES

EXPENSIVE

The biggest challenge to overcome in instigating robotic medical devices into hos-pitals is the beforehand cost it is going to take. As with any brand-new product, it arrives with a hefty price tag. Nurses and doctors will need added training, and hos-pitals will need specialized workers that will troubleshoot any issues. When more hospitals are starting to adapt to the technology and it becomes massive sales, prices will start to fall. The robotic technology is extravagant in terms of both capital costs and operating systems and will require the training of techno-scientific personnel to be responsible for the device. Those expenses may exceed any funds profited at the time. There are safety concerns corresponding to medical robots. If something goes wrong, who is to be blamed? Will it be the manufacturer, the doctor, or the worker that installed it?

Hospitals must consider the legal implications before presenting globally. These types of governing and parity will take years before landing on a final solution. Doctors will not be put out of endeavors with the development of technologies in the robotic field. Instead, these tools can help in managing tasks cautiously and sys-tematically. We should not be afraid of advancements; after all, it is what is allowing many to get the help that they need with fewer unwanted side effects [14].

PRIVACY ISSUES

Medical attention robotic devices can be accessed using supervisory devices that can give the capability of looking after the patients, documenting the required data, and communicating the required particulars through cellular networks.

Such kind of attributes can be manifested to secure elderly sick people by initi-ating indirect propinquity with their family members or hospital staff, and it will contravene patients' privacy.

Due to inadequate ample ordinance or, without monitoring, supervisory joint strategy and arrangements, the robotic devices proficiency proves to be an ultimatum to the victim's personal affairs and also to the people communicating or in contact with them. Basically, innovators in hospital and hospital management are acknowl-edged of hindmost personal-privacy business and confidentiality of data and also protection and required procedures are made aware to steer clear of such behavioral problems. For instance, at the time of evolving a nursing care robotic device, some points must be mentioned such as that the robot must not be behind the person any-where and everywhere (e.g., washroom) due to personal issues and that it is their foremost target to give elderly people the desire of safe environment [15].

RECOGNITION ISSUES

Advanced identification of a language with its dialect understanding is a highly com-plex process. Language, with its uncertainty and different meanings, is extremely tedious to process. For a machine to perform those rigorous procedures and respond to nuances is much more difficult than for a human. Humans have the ability to rec-ognize and distinguish the environment and adjust the behavior accordingly. When light prevalence changes, the discernment of the robot changes. In bright rooms, this is not much of an issue, but an assisting robot also has to function when the light of the room is dimmed.

As a football player, and as a robot, you have to be able to recognize your sur-roundings, you have to orient yourself, communicate with your teammates, make split-second decisions, and move your body accordingly. A two-legged humanoid robot of 58 cm height fitted with two camcorders, four mics, and tweeters as well as few sensors – for instance, four ultrasound and eight pressure sensors – was devel-oped. Just like its human peer, a robot must have a sense of balance, substantial sense, and power sense. Under stress, a robot's joints run hot and it loses its ability. Consequently, it needs a system that intercepts from overheating, so as to do the tasks efficiently [16].

This is one of the pivotal challenges: developing sinewy systems. In a laboratory – or in-house soccer ground – robots tend to perform pretty well. However, take them out of the lab and things get precarious: the transfer performance is still insufficient.

MOVEMENT LATENCY

One of the most notable issues with robots during surgery is the problem of latency – the duration it takes for a robot to process the commands given by a surgeon. It takes a bit of time for the computer to liaise with the robotic arms. While this is not a problem for surgeries taking place on a daily routine basis, it causes an issue for surgeons to react within a short span of time to problems that happen during the operation. With the present technology, the doctor must be in the nearest propin-quity. A long-haul challenge is to allow a surgeon to monitor the medical robotic devices, which will be used for functioning of a regular plan of action without any dependency, it also must alert the surgeon to take over during scathing, patient-specific procedures [17].

SAFETY AND SECURITY ISSUES

The wellbeing of a patient and harmlessness are the uttermost significance of a hos-pital and its management during utilization of medical robots due to participation of sick senior citizens and also youngsters. There must be a requirement for an extem-porized process, which can eradicate and may minimize safety-related omissions plus terminating unforeseeable behavior. One such peculiar thought regarding protection is to make sure that the medical robotic devices are kept safe from nefarious activities caused by hackers [18].

ETHICS

Ethics in robots has been a major challenge, which the robotics industry is cognizant of [17]. To get the awareness and emotions to various circumstances as humans do, it is really challenging to get the same in robots. Certain attributes that humans possess, machines do not, and hence acquiring a machine to get a quick reaction of such ethics eventually becomes an arduous task. Problems regarding ethics can be cited as such:

- Robots can administer tasks that are delicate to humans.
- In the occurrence of failures, humans would be held responsible.
- Reduction of employment on a large scale.
- Human freedom could be taken away completely by AI.
- Unethical usage of AI.

EMPLOYMENT ISSUES

As robots replace humans in an industry on a larger scale, it has rising concerns worldwide [19]. This could be inimical to a sector wherein the demand for human-provided nursing services is reduced. This is a sector, which is already in a setback. Employment, being an unresolved issue in such highly populated countries, eventually makes the situation unfavorable for the unemployed people or even the ones who are someday going to look for a job. Thus, when we look at the ramifications in such a situation, it clearly does present itself as a hindrance for many of them worldwide.

DIGNITY ISSUES

Humans need interaction with each other, as we are social animals by nature. By replacing humans with robots from the care environment, it leads to major issues regarding the happiness and dignity of patients. For the growth and expansion of human beings, human interaction is a necessary source. Patients enjoy such forms of interconnection when the nurse interacts and cares for them. This cannot be replaced by a robot because of its "mechanical," "pre-programmed," and thus "neutral" way to interact with patients [17]. This takes away the chief and comfortability of the patients unlike the one with the human nurse.

ATTRIBUTION OF LIABILITY ISSUES

It is impossible to accredit them responsible in case of unfavorable repercussions or glitches. Hence, it would be exceptionally intricate to accredit civil and criminal accountability to legal people who are in association with an unfavorable event brought about by a robot. Such an accountability could probably fall on people like the providers, manufacturers, technicians, and programmers. Consequently, it becomes a troublesome task for the affected patient to recognize the accountable subject. Taking into consideration the age and the vulnerability of the individuals who are commonly supposed to make use of nursing-care robots, such a task could become even infeasible [18].

BETTER POWER SOURCES

Generally, robots are energy inefficient. Enhancing the life of a battery is a paramount issue, mainly when it comes to drones and moving robots. An enlarged acquisition of these systems, thankfully, is pre-eminent to new battery technologies, which are enduring, secure, and reasonable. To build the elements of a robot with more efficiency in power, efforts are assuredly taken. Studies also show that the robots that run wirelessly in unorganized conditions, in due course, will withdraw energy from vibrations, light, and automatic movement. Research is also being done to upgrade battery technology yonder the nickel-metal hydride and lithium-ion options currently available.

CONCLUSION

At a global level, where the COVID-19 pandemic is growing at an exponential pace, the health, hygiene, and wellbeing innovations have quickly and liberally added to the management of emergencies. Various telehealth, telemedicine, teleconsultation, and telemonitoring solutions using robotics have been deployed in health centers and social care homes. However, their efficacy and effectiveness have always been a question that needs to be addressed by considering the acceptability and adoptability of the latest technologies due to potential conflicts with users' cultural, moral, and religious backgrounds. This chapter discussed the current opportunities and challenges with respect to AI-powered robots to battle COVID-19. To diminish the danger of contamination and infection, the opportunities must be utilized during this pandemic for a better future. More deliberate measures ought to be executed to guarantee that future robotic health initiatives will have a greater impact on the pandemic and meet the most key needs to facilitate the life of individuals who are at the forefront of the crisis.

Time is critical to battle COVID-19, and AI-powered robotic solutions provide the opportunity to buy time and human resources. As the COVID-19 pandemic is a worldwide health emergency, we have observed and will observe a plethora of robotic solutions. This makes a pressing requirement for strategic decision makers, policymakers, specialists, researchers, scientists, and healthcare experts to effectively implement AI-powered robotic solutions into practice without further dividing the current scenes of care. We currently call for more coordinated measures to optimally have an impact on the epidemic and to address the most vital needs to facilitate the life of individuals who are at the front line of the COVID-19 emergency [19–25].

REFERENCES

1. Zhu N, Zhang D, Wang W, Li X, Yang B, Song J, China novel coronavirus investigating and research team. A novel coronavirus from patients with pneumonia in China, 2019. *N Engl J Med* 2020 February 20;382(8): 727–733.
2. World Health Organization. Responding to community spread of COVID-19: interim guidance, 7 March 2020. https://apps.who.int/iris/handle/10665/331421 [accessed 21-10-2020].
3. Lipsitch M, Swerdlow DL, Finelli L. Defining the epidemiology of COVID-19 – studies needed. *N Engl J Med* 2020 March 26;382(13): 1194–1196.
4. From idea to PPE product in 10 days. https://www.additivemanufacturing.media/blog/post/from-idea-to-ppe-product-in-10-days-the-cool-parts-show-quarantine-edition [accessed 24-10-2020].
5. CNBC make it, Published Monday, 23 March 2020, 2:08 PM EDT Updated Monday, 23 March 2020, 2:31 PM EDT. https://www.cnbc.com/2020/03/23/video-hospital-in-china-where-covid-19-patients-treated-by-robots.html.
6. journals.sagepub.com, by MH Nguyen 2020. ISSN: 2056-3051. https://journals.sagepub.com/doi/full/10.1177/2056305120948255.
7. Luvozu, by Sam, the robotic concierge. https://luvozo.com/.
8. Nelson G, Saunders A, Neville N, Swilling B, Bondaryk J, Billings D, Lee C, Playter R, Raibert M. Petman: a humanoid robot for testing chemical protective clothing. *J Robot Soc Jpn* 2012;30(4): 372–377. https://pdfs.semanticscholar.org/69d6/fad-28347e5d47e1c47ffa3ef9d5c912f7fbd.pdf.
9. Forbes: demand for this autonomous robot is skyrocketing during pandemic May 29, by Bernard Marr, Contributor, Enterprise Tech. 2020, 12:25 am EDT. https://www.forbes.com/sites/bernardmarr/2020/05/29/demand-for-these-autonomous-delivery-robots-is-skyrocketing-during-this-pandemic/#3b69b8087f3c.
10. https://www.hansonrobotics.com/, 26 September 2020, at 21:34 (UTC).
11. Research Luxembourg: predicting the severity of COVID-19 infection. 27 April 2020. https://www.fnr.lu/predi-covid-study/.
12. Tactales tagging mechanical technologies, 04 September 2020. https://tectales.com/bionics-robotics/covid-19-robot-takes-patients-vital-signs.html.
13. The opportunities and challenges of medical robots – by Duane Boise on November 2018 in blog, Emergency medical services, medical technology. https://pt.slideshare.net/duaneboise/the-opportunities-and-challenges-of-medical-robots
14. Stahl BC, Coeckelbergh M. Ethics of healthcare robotics: towards responsible research and innovation. *Robot Autonom Syst.* 2016 December 1;86: 152–161.
15. Robots in medicine: weak knees and hard facts – blog. 05 March 2018. https://healthcare-in-europe.com/en/news/robots-in-medicine-weak-knees-hard-facts.html.
16. Robots in medicine. https://www.ncbi.nlm.nih.gov/pmc/articles/PMC6625162/#:~:text=Robots%20are%20poised%20to%20revolutionize%20the%20practice%20of%20medicine.&text=Today%2C%20medical%20robots%20are%20well, various%20surgical%20procedures%20(2).
17. Grasso C, Bioethics, Healthcare and Pharmaceuticals, Technology and Corporate Activities on The Corporate Social Responsibility and Business Ethics. Challenges and advantages of robotic nursing care: a social and ethical analysis – blog. 26 June 2018. https://corporatesocialresponsibilityblog.com/ 2018/06/26/robotic-nursing-care/
18. Crowe S. 10 Biggest challenges in Robotics. *The RobotReport*, 2 February 2018. https://www.therobotreport.com/10-biggest-challenges-in-robotics/ [accessed: 23-10-2020].

19. Sathiyanarayanan M, Rajan S. MYO Armband for physiotherapy healthcare: A case study using gesture recognition application. *2016 8th International Conference on Communication Systems and Networks (COMSNETS)*. IEEE, 2016.

20. Sathiyanarayanan M, Mulling T and Nazir B. Controlling a robot using a wearable device (MYO). *International Journal of Engineering Development and Research* 3.3 (2015).

21. Kavitha D, Murugan A, and Sathiyanarayanan M. Deep Analysis of Dementia Disorder Using Artificial Intelligence to Improve Healthcare Services. *2021 International Conference on COMmunication Systems & NETworkS (COMSNETS)*. IEEE, 2021.

22. Ganesh D et al. Automatic Health Machine for COVID-19 and Other Emergencies. *2021 International Conference on COMmunication Systems & NETworkS (COMSNETS)*. IEEE, 2021.

23. Ganesh D, Seshadri G, Sokkanarayanan S, Bose P, Rajan S, Sathiyanarayanan M. AutoImpilo: Smart Automated Health Machine using IoT to Improve Telemedicine and Telehealth. In *2020 International Conference on Smart Technologies in Computing, Electrical and Electronics (ICSTCEE)*, pp. 487-493. IEEE, 2020.

24. Ganesh D, Seshadri G, Sokkanarayanan S, Rajan S, Sathiyanarayanan M. IoT-based Google Duplex Artificial Intelligence Solution for Elderly Care. In *2019 International Conference on contemporary Computing and Informatics (IC3I)*, pp. 234–240. IEEE, 2019.

25. Rajan S, Sathiyanarayanan M, Prashant S, Prashant SB, Nataraj PL. Prevention of avoidable blindness and improving eye healthcare system in india. In *2018 10th International Conference on Communication Systems & Networks (COMSNETS)*, pp. 665–670. IEEE, 2018.

7 Analyze App Health for Ensuring Better Decision-Making and Improved Secure Outcomes

Swati Goel
Jawaharlal Nehru University

CONTENTS

INTRODUCTION

In this digital world, maintaining good health has become very much easier with the development of various health apps, which provide a holistic view of a well-balanced lifestyle by tracking the user's feelings, sleeping pattern, and eating habits to accurately monitor the health of the user. Mobile health apps (mhealth) is a rising technological trend especially among younger generations because of some factors like convenience, education, encouraging a healthy lifestyle, and so on. Accessing mhealth on just one click is very much easier compared to visiting a hospital for daily routine checkups, which is both time and cost consuming. Easy accessibility of these health apps is one of the reasons for the rising popularity of these apps. Healthcare apps are a boon not only to doctors but also to medical staff. They have many advantages; they provide opportunistic models for handling emergency situations, they can

130   Robotic Technologies

be accessed in far remote areas, and many more uncountable benefits are provided to stakeholders; but these apps have some serious privacy and security issues like data security, lack of app-specific protocols, security issues in mobile devices, lack of regulation, and so on. [1]. So, in this chapter, we will analyze healthcare apps on various parameters like security, reliability of outcome, and trustworthiness so that an informed improved decision can be taken, which will also be secure.

Mobile health applications (mhealth apps) are basically programs written on software that provide health-related information on mobile phones and tablets [2]. The usage of mhealth apps is increasing rapidly because of the rising demand and supply of smartphones, including Google's Android platform and Apple's iPhone. Mhealth apps can be used by clients from everywhere, no matter whether they are using it from their home or workplace. The majority of users of these apps use them for self-monitoring purposes like checking blood sugar levels, blood pressure, calories intake, and so on. Mhealth apps are one of the different fields that have used innovative ideas and concepts and have expanded exponentially and progressing continuously. Taking the data into account, Apple iOS App store [3] has approximately more than 31,000 apps that are related to health, medicine, and fitness; on the other side, Android's Google play store [3] has more than 16,000 medical and healthcare apps [3]. Clinicians and patients are adopting these mhealth apps on a large scale and they have become part of their daily activities, but being unaware of various security and privacy concerns associated with these mobile apps, they are taking risk with lives of humankind.

Healthcare applications are efficient in maintaining a proper balance between easy usability and user burden [4]. Usability can be defined as the level of difficulty experienced by the user while using these mhealth apps [5]. User burden is not clearly defined in the literature, but from our understanding, user burden can be the mental resources needed to accomplish a particular task. These apps are designed to be user-centric for tracking their health conditions and accessing these apps requires a lot of efforts from the app users. Hence, from this, we can conclude that these healthcare apps increase user burden to some extent, making many users drop the use of these apps. Therefore, if developers want to promote these user-centric health tracking mobile apps, they need to focus on enhancing the app's usability while simultaneously concentrating on lowering the user burden [4].

Healthcare facilities worldwide face numerous challenges and the management of medicines is one of the prominent ones. By adopting these mhealth apps, a patient's medicine management journey can be made simpler [6], starting from booking an appointment, consultation, decision-making, information acquisition, and monitoring and management in day-to-day life. These mhealth apps have a huge potential in overcoming the barriers of healthcare system by providing low cost, high-quality, and evidence-based health information to their users by following standard guidelines or protocols via behavioral change models [7]. For strengthening healthcare facilities globally, there must be a provision of universal healthcare system for which developers need to work on three factors, namely enhancing quality, accessibility of basic healthcare facilities, and cost optimization. Literature regarding the efficiency of mhealth apps is still evolving and many researchers are trying to understand the reliability of these apps. Because of the lack of formal procedures and evidence-based clinical research, there is some reluctance from healthcare providers in prescribing mhealth apps to their patients.

Healthcare apps have some privacy concerns such as the data of patients, physicians, and primary healthcare workers need to be secure. One of the most important aspects in building a secure healthcare system is to prevent unauthorized people from accessing sensitive and confidential data [8]. Sensitive health-related information of patients can be accessed through wireless technologies raising various security and privacy-associated issues in the usage of these apps and these issues raise many questions on the credibility of these mhealth apps. In order to make these apps secure, users should have the choice of sharing their data but mostly they are unaware of the amount of leakage of information that takes place via their mobile phones. Hence, there is a need to analyze the available health apps by taking into account the various privacy concerns so that a better decision can be made and the final result delivered will be more secured.

This chapter is organized as follows: the "Machine Learning in Healthcare Applications" section discusses about machine learning in healthcare apps. The "Privacy and Security Issues in HealthCare Apps" section discusses the aspects of privacy and security-related issues. The framed research questions that have been discussed are explained in the "Research Questions" section. The uses and benefits of healthcare apps are elaborated in the "Healthcare Apps: Uses and Benefits" section. The decision-making process is discussed in the "Decision-Making in HealthCare Apps" section, and finally, the issues and challenges of healthcare apps are discussed in the "Issues and Challenges in HealthCare Applications" section.

MACHINE LEARNING IN HEALTHCARE APPLICATIONS

There can be many uses of machine learning (ML) in healthcare applications, but the major advantage is the processing of a very large amount of dataset, which is not possible by manual processing, and then transforming the fetched analysis of data into valuable insight, which can be further used by doctors for providing good quality healthcare, which ultimately gives secure outcomes, satisfying the patients and increasing the trust of patients on these mhealth apps. ML plays a crucial role in decision-making by training the system to analyze pictures, identifying abnormalities, and finding out critical areas that need special attention, thus improving the efficiency, accuracy, and reliability of all these processes.

The performance of healthcare can be improved through ML including computer-aided diagnosis, image registration, medical image segmentation, image annotation, guiding through a medical image, and so on where a single error can prove to be very harmful [9]. For lowering the price of healthcare, ML can provide a solution and it can also be used as a tool for improving communication between a doctor and a patient [10]. If ML is applied effectively, it can be used by physicians in making perfect diagnoses and prescribing good quality medication to their patients, which enhances the patient's health in optimized cost of treatment. Better decisions can be taken by physicians by employing ML, which takes care of everything about the health of a patient behind the scenes and prompts the doctor to take more informed decision.

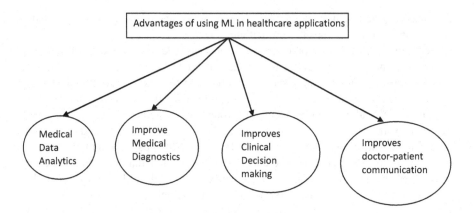

FIGURE 7.1 Benefits of ML in healthcare apps.

Doctors find it very challenging to draw conclusions from the patient dataset as datasets are sometimes incomplete, incorrect, and not exact [11]. Thomas H. Davenport writes in the Wall Street Journal, "Humans can typically create one or two good models a week (while) machine learning can create thousands of models a week." Figure 7.1 shows the major benefits of using ML in the healthcare sector.

ROBOTICS IN HEALTHCARE

The use of robots in the healthcare industry can completely transform the health-care sector, which will support doctors and nurses by automatizing several tasks and will also assist in patient care. However, it is also true that expert doctors cannot be replaced by anything though robots will only serve as a helping hand to doctors to improve the efficiency of work. Some of the benefits of using robots in the healthcare industry are given below:

   i. Improved accuracy
  ii. Remote treatment
 iii. Complementing human abilities
 iv. Precise diagnosis

PRIVACY AND SECURITY ISSUES IN HEALTHCARE APPS

Mhealth applications have become so much popular among patients for connecting with health advisors or chronic care assistants. The reason behind the high demand of these apps is their easy accessibility and these apps provide a single platform for patients' healthcare journey, starting from booking an appointment to proper treat-ment of a patient's disease. These apps gather a huge amount of patient data based on varying health behavior, which raises privacy and security concerns over the usage of these apps in the case of major clinical levels, across the health network. These apps not only share data with the doctors (healthcare professionals) but also in patient's

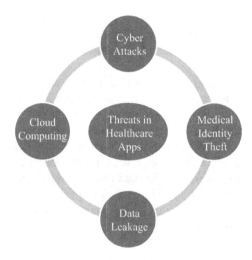

FIGURE 7.2   Prominent threats in healthcare apps.

relationship circle like family, friends, colleagues, patient's insurance company, and so on, which is a critical problem with these apps [12]. These apps also have the ability to share the data with third-party organizations such as advertisers or payment service providers, which puts the confidential user data in a high risk [8].

The study of author McCarthy shows that out of many free apps available, only 25% provide a privacy policy to their users [13]. Mobile applications have become a new target of hackers because most users keep their sensitive data in mobile devices, which makes mheatlh apps highly vulnerable to various security attacks. Threats related to malware, data interception, device loss, and tampering occur frequently in mobile environment [12]. Figure 7.2 shows the major threats related to healthcare applications.

In order to improve the quality and efficiency and to reduce cost and medical errors of healthcare services, providers are adopting digital technologies like personal health records (PHR), medical practice management software (MPMS), and many other digital components. To avoid data leakage and cyber attacks in healthcare apps, developers have to go beyond traditional cryptographic mechanisms and adopt some novel techniques such as control theory, game theory, and other disciplines.

RESEARCH QUESTIONS

The main aim of this research is to collect and investigate all of the credible and effective studies that have examined privacy and security issues in healthcare apps. To achieve this goal and identify the methods that have been used by various researchers in their studies, the following research questions (RQs) are raised.

RQ1: Identify the stages where privacy policy has been implemented in healthcare apps. Are there any standard guidelines followed by developers of these healthcare apps?

Motivation: This question allows us to get an overview of key areas where most developers have implemented privacy policy in these apps to make their app more secure and confidential and how we can improve the privacy policy implementation by making it standardized.

Discussion: Apps belonging to the healthcare category have been selected from the Google play store for the purpose of understanding RQ1 as shown in Table 7.1. It is clearly visible from Table 7.1 that the stages where privacy is implemented in various apps are not uniform, but data collection, data sharing, and data processing are the areas where most developers have implemented privacy features. Privacy policy generally explains the procedure involved in the collection of data and sharing, usage, and protection of personal information of end-users. For making the app reliable, privacy policy has to be implemented in a specific way because it shows the commitment of the app toward the privacy of data of the app's end-users. Hence, we propose specific steps for providing privacy in healthcare applications, which are as follows:

Step 1: Apps should take consent from the users for collection of their sensitive personal information.

Step 2: Users are required to accept the Term of use of the app in order to access the app's services.

Step 3: For sharing the user's data with a third party, the user's consent must be taken.

Step 4: Apps should have the authority of discontinuing app services to those users who have provided inaccurate information.

Step 5: Apps should have the provision where users can e-mail to the admin of the app if they want to cancel their account or discontinue receiving non-essential e-mails.

Step 6: User's credit card/debit card details are transacted on secure sites of approved payment gateways.

Step 7: Apps should not allow storing any personal information of the users.

For making healthcare apps more secure, the above-proposed steps need to be incorporated in the apps, which will make the privacy policy standardized and it will also enhance the trust of the users in the app.

HEALTHCARE APPS: USES AND BENEFITS

Healthcare technology is useful in all medical fields and it is helpful for both patients and doctors as shown in Table 7.2. These apps are more important for patients who have some serious disease and require continuous monitoring of their health condition to have a permanent check on their health. The wide usage of these apps has transformed the communication pattern between doctors and patients. Patient's data collection and retrieval of information such as medical history, prescriptions, lab results, scans, and so on have become much easier with the help of these apps [14]. The healthcare system is distributed in different areas such as clinics, operation theaters, labs, and so on [15].

TABLE 7.1

Apps in the Healthcare Category from Google Play Store

S. No.	App Name	Description	Where Privacy Policy is Implemented?
1	Apollo247	This app ensures 24*7 hours doctor availability within 15 minutes of booking an appointment and medicines will be delivered at the doorstep of patients in less than 3 hours	Data collection, storage, processing and disclosure, and transfer of user's personal information
2	Medlife-India's largest E-Health Platform	This app provides high-quality online medicine; doctor consultation and diagnostic tests can be booked online	Data collection, processing, personal information usage
3	Aayu	This app provides treatment of almost all types of health-related diseases from specialized doctors at affordable prices	Data collection, data processing, data sharing, legal bases
4	1mg-Online medical store & healthcare app	This app provides users the facility of viewing medicine information, online buying of medicines, booking lab tests and health checkups, and so on	Data collection, data retention, data sharing
5	PharmEasy-Online Medicine Ordering App	This app allows ordering medicines online, booking health packages and diagnostic tests online, and so on	Data collection, data sharing
6	Netmeds-India's trusted Online pharmacy App	This app allows free access to health information to their users, consulting best doctors online, booking lab tests online, and so on	Data collection, data usage
7	MFine-consult doctors online and book health tests	This app allows users to talk to a doctor to get informed doctor consultation, timely medicine reminders will be sent on the user's phone, and so on	Data collection, data receipt, storage, usage, processing, sharing
8	Practo	This app allows users to consult and chat with a doctor online, users can buy affordable health plans, and so on	Data collection, usage, sharing, disclosure, and protection of personal information
9	Blood Pressure Tracker-BP tracker-BP Logger	This app maintains BP levels and sugar levels with many in-built functionalities like measurement analysis, graphs, comprehensive reports, and so on	Data collection, data sharing, data processing
10	Wellness Forever	This app allows users to order medicines online at any time and there is no minimum order limit in this app, which makes it affordable to everyone	Data collection, data sharing, data processing

TABLE 7.2

HealthCare Apps Uses and Benefits

Healthcare Professionals	Patients
1. Improved accuracy	1. Access online health tips
2. Improved efficiency	2. Access cloud service
3. Increase productivity	3. Quality care
4. Allows taking informed clinical decision	4. Patients will feel more secure by reading the privacy guidelines of the app
5. Reduce complexity	5. Accessible from everywhere
6. Proactive decisions can be taken according to the patient's condition	6. Can easily search for a specialized health practitioner
7. Easy access and update of health record	7. Medication plans and can fix intake reminders
8. Continuous monitoring of patient health condition	8. Increased patient engagement

Common Uses and Benefits

1. Effective in time management by scheduling meetings and appointments
2. Better communication between doctors and patients
3. Easily accessible even from far remote areas
4. Medical education and training

Mhealth apps are also getting a lot of attention because of their ability to provide public heath surveillance, being helpful in community data gathering and monitoring health of disabled individuals [16]. We have found some relevant literature review in this study, which successfully highlighted the use of mobile apps to support tele-medicines and remote healthcare [17]. Due to the large potential of the mhealth apps, the healthcare system is changing around the world drastically. Figure 7.3 shows the major benefits of mobile technology in the healthcare system.

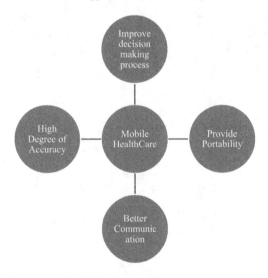

FIGURE 7.3   Benefits of mobile technology in the healthcare system.

While making the mhealth apps, developers have to consider the following three things carefully:

1. Confidential policy
2. Getting approval from regulatory bodies
3. App performance testing criteria

Mhealth apps contain a lot of personal data of patients; hence, it is very necessary for the developers of the app to protect sensitive information of the patients by following confidential policy. In addition to this, patients should also know that their personal data are safe within the app and it can be deleted anytime if they think it is necessary. Also, the developer of the app has to perform load testing to ensure the accessibility and reliability of the app.

DECISION-MAKING IN HEALTHCARE APPS

Healthcare apps have transformed numerous factors that deal with the making of decisions in the healthcare field by healthcare professionals [18]. Several health apps make smartphones invaluable tools that support clinical decision-making at the point of care [19]. While practicing evidence-based medicine, the quality factor is very important to maintain because clinicians may always not seek an answer to every clinical question after the clinical encounter [20]. In the medical field, decision-making is one of the complex processes in terms of many factors such as possibilities of outcomes and the quantity of information that can be processed.

There are many ways in which decision-making procedures for healthcare professionals can be studied. One of that is by using the cognitive load approach [21], where quality of healthcare service and decision-making provided to patients are affected by cognitive overload. For improving the process of decision-making, the focus of healthcare workers has to be on the most important information first, information color-coding, and presenting information to healthcare practitioners in a multimodal way can improve the cognitive-load. Mhealth apps are designed by developers in such a way that they support shared decision-making in diagnostics and treatment [22].

There are many health problems in which choosing the best course of action is difficult because of the probabilistic nature of treatment and diagnosis [23]. Shared decision-making can be defined as the procedure that allows both patients and their healthcare providers to take mutual decisions. By taking the best available scientific result as well as their choice [24] into consideration, patients should be well aware about the critical role performed by them in the decision-making process and efficient tools must be provided to them, which help them in understanding the performance and consequence of their taken decisions. The shared decision-making procedure allows one to select the optimal decision. The usage of these apps is cost effective and it will reduce the load on paper-based documents for both patients and doctors.

This shared decision-making is proving to be very potential as it has numerous advantages in the healthcare system, but it has some disadvantages also, like it may undermine the quality of physician–patient relationships [25]. Currently, in mhealth apps, there are some regulations, which say that poor quality of health care and incorrect information can misguide patients and can adversely affect their health.

ISSUES AND CHALLENGES IN HEALTHCARE APPLICATIONS

Healthcare apps have proved to be an effective tool in improving accessibility to healthcare services, making an informed healthcare decision, and increased self-awareness among patients regarding basic healthcare. These apps have some issues and challenges and the major ones are shown in Figures 7.4 and 7.5 respectively. One of the critical issues in healthcare apps is Health literacy [26]. Health literacy has been defined in a study [27] as "the degree to which individuals have the capacity to obtain, process and understand basic health information and services they need to make appropriate health decisions.". The success rate of these apps depends on the level of awareness among patients regarding health while a low health literacy rate will remain a problem. Hence, mHealth apps have "to be developed using best practice strategies to present information in ways that are understandable to each of the intended audience [27].". In addition, not every individual has sufficient digital knowledge to operate the mhealth apps so usability is another key issue in these apps. Affording high priced smart phones is also the barrier in accessing high quality health services of these apps. A gradual increase in the number of these apps requires their developers to increase their focus on risk assessment. Interoperability can be defined as the ability of various medical systems to interact with each other and exchange patients' health-related information in a protected environment. Interoperability plays an important role in the making

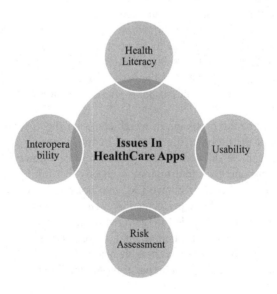

FIGURE 7.4 Major issues in healthcare apps.

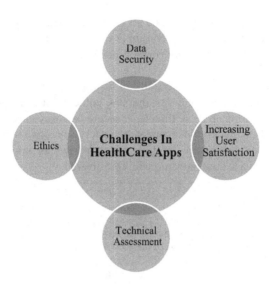

FIGURE 7.5 Major challenges in healthcare apps.

of accurate health decisions by doctors because it makes sure that data will be available to doctors on time.

There are four major challenges, which need to be taken care of while developing these apps as shown in Figure 7.5. Data security is one of the grave concerns to healthcare organizations. While exchanging or data sharing patient's sensitive information over wireless communication, there is a possibility of data leakage. Hence, to overcome these challenges, developers have to establish a mobile storage and retrieval system, which will be threat proof. An application has to be designed in a user-friendly manner, and then only it will be possible to gain confidence of the users on these apps. The HealthCare IT infrastructure is already complex with multiple layers of systems, devices, applications, and network. Therefore, technical assessment is highly necessary in these apps by integrating mobility by placing a new layer of complexity. There is one more important challenge in these apps, which is ensuring ethics, which comprise privacy, trust, and responsibility for errors [28]. Medical errors can lead to deaths also. Hence, guidelines have to be defined for making the person accountable of errors.

CONCLUSION

A secure healthcare environment is needed to build trust among patients, which is possible when both users and developers adopt standard guidelines. The fundamental level of quality and safety has to be ensured in these apps by hardcore evaluation, validation, and the development of best-practice standard for medical apps [29]. Healthcare apps are very useful in improving patient safety and reducing medication errors. Emerging technologies like artificial intelligence and ML are affecting the healthcare sector to a greater extent and accessing a basic quality healthcare service is the human necessity. To gain the consumer confidence and trust in these medical apps, extensive and transparent information has to be provided on the web page of the app [30].

Cybersecurity threats occur frequently in healthcare apps. Hence, developers of these apps must continuously monitor the new vulnerabilities in order to take precautionary steps to mitigate these threats. A secure two-way messaging channel has to be established between providers and patients for accessing the hospital workflow management. Hence, these apps, if designed properly, can improve the decision-making process and a secure outcome will be delivered.

REFERENCES

1. R. Adhikari, D. Richards, and K. Scott, "Security and privacy issues related to the use of mobile health apps," *Proceedings of the 25th Australasian Conference on Information Systems ACIS 2014, no. Schulke 2013*, Auckland, New Zealand, 2014.
2. A. Tkachenko, "Media Contact: Remedy health media receives top merits from industry leaders," pp. 2013–2014, 2014.
3. B. Martínez-Pérez, I. de la Torre-Díez, and M. López-Coronado, "Privacy and security in mobile health apps: A review and recommendations," *J. Med. Syst.*, vol. 39, no. 1, 2015, doi: 10.1007/s10916-014-0181-3.
4. S. D. Birkhoff and S. C. Smeltzer, "Perceptions of smartphone user-centered mobile health tracking apps across various chronic illness populations: An integrative review," *J. Nurs. Scholarsh.*, vol. 49, no. 4, pp. 371–378, 2017, doi: 10.1111/jnu.12298.
5. J. Cho, D. Park, and H. E. Lee, "Cognitive factors of using health apps: Systematic analysis of relationships among health consciousness, health information orientation, eHealth literacy, and health app use efficacy," *J. Med. Internet Res.*, vol. 16, no. 5, pp. 1–10, 2014, doi: 10.2196/jmir.3283.
6. J. Car, W. S. Tan, Z. Huang, P. Sloot, and B. D. Franklin, "eHealth in the future of medications management: Personalisation, monitoring and adherence," *BMC Med.*, vol. 15, no. 1, pp. 1–9, 2017, doi: 10.1186/s12916-017-0838-0.
7. B. Fogg, "A behavior model for persuasive design," *ACM Int. Conf. Proc. Ser.*, vol. 350, 2009, doi: 10.1145/1541948.1541999.
8. B. H. Sampat and B. Prabhakar, "Privacy risks and security threats in mHealth apps," *J. Int. Technol. Inf. Manag.*, vol. 26, no. 4, pp. 126–153, 2017.
9. G. Winter, "Machine learning in healthcare," *Br. J. Heal. Care Manag.*, vol. 25, no. 2, pp. 100–101, 2019, doi: 10.12968/bjhc.2019.25.2.100.
10. R. Bhardwaj, A. R. Nambiar, and D. Dutta, "A study of machine learning in healthcare," *Proc. Int. Comput. Softw. Appl. Conf.*, vol. 2, pp. 236–241, 2017, doi: 10.1109/COMPSAC.2017.164.
11. G. D. Magoulas and A. Prentza, "Machine learning in medical applications," *Lecturer Notes in Computer Science (including Subseries Lecturer Notes in Artificial Intellegent Lecture Notes in Bioinformatics), vol. 2049 LNAI*, pp. 300–307, 2001, doi: 10.1007/3-540-44673-7_19.
12. A. K. Jain and D. Shanbhag, "Addressing security and privacy risks in mobile applications," *IT Prof.*, vol. 14, no. 5, pp. 28–33, 2012, doi: 10.1109/MITP.2012.72.
13. M. McCarthy, "Experts warn on data security in health and fitness apps.," *BMJ*, vol. 347, no. September, p. 57216, 2013, doi: 10.1136/bmj.f5600.
14. C. Lee Ventola, "Mobile devices and apps for health care professionals: Uses and benefits," *Pharmacol. Ther.*, vol. 39, no. 5, pp. 356–364, 2014.

15. A. S. M. Mosa, I. Yoo, and L. Sheets, "A systematic review of healthcare applications for smartphones," *BMC Med. Inform. Decis. Mak.*, vol. 12, no. 1, 2012, doi: 10.1186/1472-6947-12-67.

16. M. N. K. Boulos, S. Wheeler, C. Tavares, and R. Jones, "How smartphones are changing the face of mobile and participatory healthcare: An overview, with example from eCAALYX," *Biomed. Eng. Online*, vol. 10, no. 1, p. 24, 2011, doi: 10.1186/1475-925X-10-24.

17. J. A. Blaya, H. S. F. Fraser, and B. Holt, "E-health technologies show promise in developing countries," *Health Aff.*, vol. 29, no. 2, pp. 244–251, 2010, doi: 10.1377/hlthaff.2009.0894.

18. S. Wallace, M. Clark, and J. White, "'It's on my iPhone': Attitudes to the use of mobile computing devices in medical education, a mixed-methods study," *BMJ Open*, vol. 2, no. 4, pp. 1–7, 2012, doi: 10.1136/bmjopen-2012-001099.

19. P. Divall, J. Camosso-Stefinovic, and R. Baker, "The use of personal digital assistants in clinical decision making by health care professionals: A systematic review," *Health Informatics J.*, vol. 19, no. 1, pp. 16–28, 2013, doi: 10.1177/1460458212446761.

20. S. Mickan, J. K. Tilson, H. Atherton, N. W. Roberts, and C. Heneghan, "Evidence of effectiveness of health care professionals using handheld computers: A scoping review of systematic reviews," *J. Med. Internet Res.*, vol. 15, no. 10, pp. 1–9, 2013, doi: 10.2196/jmir.2530.

21. J. Sweller, "Cognitive load during problem solving: Effects on learning – Sweller – 2010 – Cognitive science – Wiley Online Library," *Cogn. Sci.*, vol. 285, pp. 257–285, 1988, doi: 10.1207/s15516709cog1202_4.

22. S. A. Rahimi, M. Menear, H. Robitaille, and F. Légaré, "Are mobile health applications useful for supporting shared decision making in diagnostic and treatment decisions?," *Glob. Health Action*, vol. 10, no. 3, 2017, doi: 10.1080/16549716.2017.1332259.

23. H. J. Van Duijn, M. M. Kuyvenhoven, H. M. Tiebosch, F. G. Schellevis, and T. J. M. Verheij, "Diagnostic labelling as determinant of antibiotic prescribing for acute respiratory tract episodes in general practice," *BMC Fam. Pract.*, vol. 8, pp. 1–5, 2007, doi: 10.1186/1471-2296-8-55.

24. M. J. Barry and S. Edgman-Levitan, "Shared decision making – The pinnacle of patient-centered care," *N. Engl. J. Med.*, vol. 366, no. 9, pp. 780–781, 2012, doi: 10.1056/NEJMp1109283.

25. W. C. Hsu "Utilization of a cloud-based diabetes management program for insulin initiation and titration enables collaborative decision making between healthcare providers and patients," *Diabetes Technol. Ther.*, vol. 18, no. 2, pp. 59–67, 2016, doi: 10.1089/dia.2015.0160.

26. S. Jusoh, "A survey on trend, opportunities and challenges of mHealth apps," *Int. J. Interact. Mob. Technol.*, vol. 11, no. 6, pp. 73–85, 2017, doi: 10.3991/ijim.v11i6.7265.

27. US Department of Health and Human Services, "Healthy People 2010: General data issues," pp. 1–56, 2010.

28. G. Bhutkar, J. Karande, and M. Dhore, "Major challenges with mobile healthcare applications," *Br. J. Healthc. Comput. Inf. Manag.*, 2009, [Online]. Available: http://www.bjhcim.co.uk/features/2009/909004.htm.

29. R. B. Jones, M. N. K. Boulos, S. Wheeler, C. Tavares, and R. Jones, "How smartphones are changing the face of mobile and participatory healthcare : an overview, with example from eCAALYX," *Biomed. Eng. Online*, vol. 10, no. 1, pp. 1–14, 2011, doi: 10.1186/1475-925X-10-24.

30. U. V. Albrecht, O. Pramann, and U. Von Jan, "Synopsis for health apps: Transparency for trust and decision making," In *Social Media and Mobile Technologies for Healthcare*, pp. 94–108, 2014, doi: 10.4018/978-1-4666-6150-9.ch007.

8 Intelligent Robots in the Disease Recovery Process Using a Whale Optimization-Based Feature Selection and Classification Model

Denis A. Pustokhin
State University of Management

Irina V. Pustokhina
Plekhanov Russian University of Economics

Eswaran Perumal and K. Shankar
Alagappa University

CONTENTS

INTRODUCTION

A robot is an active agent that connects with the real-time environment and regularly works under considerate and uncontrolled conditions. While robots have fixed and re-prepared capacities, they ought to have the option to adjust or extend to complete new and valuable assignments. It is yet a challenging factor to utilize robots with pre-assembled aptitudes and the capacity to get new abilities. Consequently, applying deep learning (DL) to the robots leads to several research questions [1]. Deep reinforcement learning (DRL) has been effectively employed in different working environments for learning complex courses of action through huge quantity observations, e.g., pictures. Robots can, along these lines, be utilized to do everyday activities, for example, washing garments, cooking, and cleaning. Applying DL ways to deal with genuine humanoid robots, nonetheless, stays a critical test, as customary DRL methods include countless learning instances. DL and artificial intelligence (AI) have gotten significant interest in the course of the most recent couple of years [2,3]. These advances are changing different applications like medical services, computer vision, design acknowledgment, robots, self-driving vehicles, programmed machine interpretation, and so on [4–9].

Compared with all other applications, the medical sector is an effective and significant field. DL stores a massive amount of patient details such as patient personal details, medical information, and insurance data, in a neural network (NN) for developing effective simulation outcomes [10,11]. Here, disease prediction models an effective role in people's routine life, which is assumed to be more essential in educational sectors [12]. In the case of healthcare system, data mining (DM) models play an important role in disease prediction. The processes involved in the healthcare sector are shown in Figure 8.1. Disease prediction systems (DPSs), with various DM approaches, have gained maximum attention. The prominently applied DM schemes include a single-layer perceptron (SLP) classifier that has been applied in detecting diverse types of diseases. Here, AI and machine learning (ML) methods are combined to mitigate the healthcare problems in real-time scenarios. Recently, NN and corresponding applications are employed significantly in various domains, which guide clinical analysis. NN ensembles improvise the simplification abilities of the learning mechanism using predefined NN and combine the attained simulation outcomes. Developers have executed ML approaches globally to resist COVID-19,

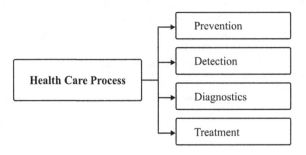

FIGURE 8.1   Process in healthcare.

cardiac disorder, breast cancer, and so on. Even though the attained prediction results are effective, further enhancement is essential by enhanced feature engineering. The different sources of medical data are given in Figure 8.2.

Loey et al. [13] showed a new prediction DL-relied generative adversarial network (GAN) scheme for COVID-19 X-ray datasets. The major strategy of the newly developed method is to consider X-ray images as input. Virus prediction is carried out using the GAN DL classifier. Hence, the introduced approach limits the complexity, storage application, and duration. Zhou et al. [14] presented an automated COVID-19 computed tomography segmentation method under the application of U-net spatial as well as channel attention structure. U-net is composed of two components, namely encoder and decoder, and it has been employed for clinical image segmentation of COVID-19. Contextual correlations are found in a region of interest (ROI) using spatial and channel concentrations for better experience in segmentation. Hence, the newly developed method is processed on minimal datasets. Ghoshal et al. [15] utilized a Bayesian convolutional neural network (BCNN) DL dataset for predicting coronavirus uncertainty and interpretability (COVID-19) and X-ray dataset to enhance the diagnosing function. Evaluation of uncertainty in DL outcomes is highly scalable in disease detection, which results in making negative assumptions.

Nilashi et al. [16] deployed a new method for disease forecasting using a clustering approach. In this approach, classification and regression trees (CART) have been employed to make fuzzy-based rules. Also, the simulation outcomes have implied that the model applied significantly enhances the accuracy of disease detections. Chuan et al. [17] used privacy-preserving disease prediction (PPDP). In this approach, patient's historical clinical data are outsourced and encrypted, which are further employed for training prediction schemes. Hence, the risk in diagnosing disease with a medical survey is assessed according to the prediction approaches. Chen et al. [18] developed a computational model of ensemble method for predicting microRNA (miRNA) infection. These examinations are processed on three main tumors. On the other hand, kidney cancer, prostate cancer, and lymphoma of top ranked and detected miRNAs are developed by present experimental outcomes as depicted by hybrid approach for miRNA-disease association prediction (HAMDA).

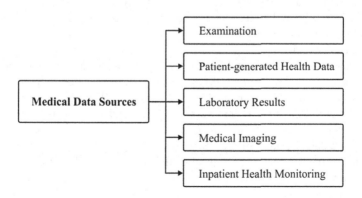

FIGURE 8.2   Sources of medical data.

Parisot et al. [19] recommended a methodological estimation of generic architecture, such as non-imagery as well as imaging data named graphic convolutional networks (GCNs), which employed brain studies in massive populations. Also, the extensive evaluation finds the issues involved in every element for disease detection and assessing the baselines. Weng et al. [20] developed a technology for investigating the function of various classifiers and a single classification model is considered as an ensemble classifier (EC). Statistical tests have been performed for assessing the functional differentiation among various classifiers. Kumar et al. [21] formulated a novel approach for diabetes prediction. Moreover, a new classifier that relies on fuzzy rules is developed for disease prediction. Hence, experiments are processed under the application of actual health records gathered from various hospitals. Luo et al. [22] established a novel approach for an miRNA-association of diseases dependant on a graphic regularization framework (MDAGRF). The working function of this approach is not susceptible to specific constraints. The MDAGRF is applicable in gaining enhanced predictive results for specific infections. Sengupta and Asit [23] deployed a technique that relied on particle swarm optimization (PSO) and association rule mining (ARM).

Initially, the fuzzy logic system (FLS) was presented in Ref. [16], which is an efficient method used for disease analysis, and it yields best outcomes by noise ignorance. Following this, PPDP was employed in Ref. [17], which provides enhanced privacy protection with minimum processing complexity; however, there is a need for significant PPDP approaches. Additionally, the HAMDA model was developed in a study [18] that offers better function and enhanced prediction capability. But, it requires best biological observations in future advancements. Similarly, the GCN method was applied in a study [19], which provided better accuracy and examined different labels. Furthermore, EC was utilized in a study [20], which offered the best accuracy and is cheaper with massive advantages; hence, the external verification of EC has to be evaluated in the future. Next, the fuzzy rule was employed in a study [21], which gave maximum specificity and security, but, the cryptographic methods have to be considered. Moreover, the MDAGRF is considered in Ref. [22], which is capable of generating the best disease prediction results and consistent information; however, it is embedded with noisy data. Additionally, the PSO approach was recommended in Ref. [23] that generates effective results and maximum efficiency. Thus, it needs contemplation on increased data with distinct feature sets. Finally, a defined constraint has to be assumed to improvise the disease prediction effectively in projected research.

This chapter projects an intelligent robot in the disease discovery process using a whale optimization algorithm (WOA)-based feature selection (FS) with a fuzzy rule-based classifier (FRBC), named WOA-FRBC. The WOA-FRBC model involves three distinct stages, namely preprocessing, FS, and classification. Besides, the WOA-based FS process is applied to extract a useful set of features from the provided preprocessed data. Besides, the FRBC model is employed for classification purposes, which determine the proper class label of the applied data. To investigate the proficient results of the WOA-FRBC model, several experiments were performed. The experimental outcomes show that the WOA-FRBC model has a better diagnostic outcome than those of the earlier techniques.

THE WOA-FRBC MODEL

Figure 8.3 shows the working principle of the WOA-FRBC model. The input medical data are initially preprocessed by the robots to enhance the quality of the dataset. Then, the WOA-FS algorithm gets executed to extract an optimal feature subset. Following this, the FRBC technique is employed to identify the existence of the disease and determine the class label.

THE WOA-FS MODEL

Here, WOA is mainly applied for the FS process. WOA is defined as a stochastic population-relied method triggered by the bubble-net feeding nature of humpback whales [24]. At this point, swimming in a '6'-shaped path is highly essential. Also, WOA is operated on two primary levels: exploration and exploitation. In the case of exploration, a whale identifies the prey in random fashion, whereas in the second level, the model of encircling a prey and spiral bubble-net attacking is followed.

A feature subset is assumed as a location of a whale in WOA. The subset is composed of N features. Under the application of minimum features in all solutions, the classification accuracy attained is considerable. A solution is verified based on the presented fitness function, which depends upon two major objectives: a solution's accuracy accomplished by a DNN classifier and count of selected features from a solution. In a population, optimal solution is pointed as X^* (prey). The key objective

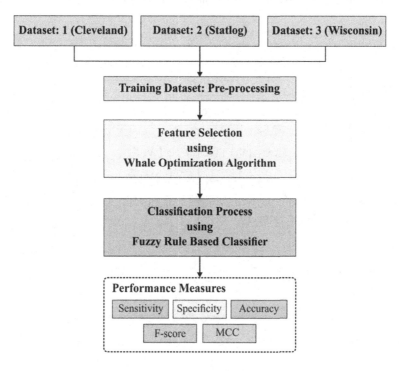

FIGURE 8.3   Process involved in the proposed model.

in WOA is followed to the greater extent. In all iterations, a solution is upgraded with the position relied on bubble-net attacking as well as exploration for prey. The bubble-net attacking is reflected by selecting the shrinking encircling framework (Eq.8.2) and spiral model (Eq. 8.6) for enhancing the solution position (whales). The possible position of a solution in WOA is shown in Figure 8.4.

The task of surrounding a prey is evaluated in Eqs. (8.1) and (8.2):

$$\vec{D} = \left| \vec{C} \cdot \vec{X}^*(t) - \vec{X}(t) \right| \tag{8.1}$$

$$\vec{X}(t+1) = \vec{X}^*(t) - \vec{A} \cdot \vec{D} \tag{8.2}$$

where t implies the recent iteration, X^* denotes the optimal solution, X means the current solution, $\|$ indicates the proper value, and $\cdot$ signifies an element by element multiplication. The coefficient vectors A and C are measured by the given function.

$$\vec{A} = 2\vec{a} \cdot \vec{r} - \vec{r} \tag{8.3}$$

$$\vec{C} = 2 \cdot \vec{r} \tag{8.4}$$

where a is reduced linearly from 2 to 0 and r implies a vector from [0,1]. To increase the searching ability of WOA, despite requiring solutions to identify randomly based optimal positions, the arbitrarily decided solution has been used to

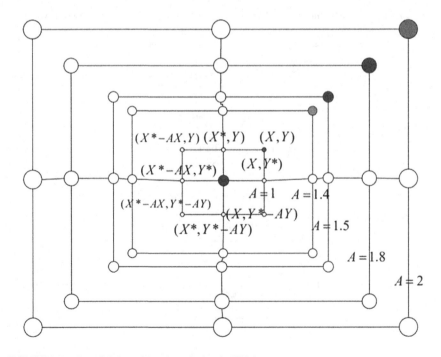

FIGURE 8.4 Possible location of a solution in WOA.

upgrade the position. Hence, a vector A with random values that is maximum than 1 or minimum than −1 has been applied to the developed solution from the best search agent, which is described in Eqs. (8.5) and (8.6).

$$\vec{D} = \left| \vec{C}.\overrightarrow{X_{\text{rand}}} - \vec{X} \right| \qquad (8.5)$$

$$\vec{X}(t+1) = \overrightarrow{X_{\text{rand}}} - \vec{A} \cdot \vec{D} \qquad (8.6)$$

where $\overrightarrow{X_{\text{rand}}}$ denotes a random whale decided from a recent population. Based on the application of the shrinking encircling principle, an effective tradeoff between exploitation and exploration is required. The random vector A that exists among the measures of >1 or <1 is applied. If $A > 1$, then exploration is performed for exploring the neighbor of the randomly selected solution, and the neighbor of the best solution is applied in $A < 1$. Hence, the above-defined operation is repeated till reaching the termination condition.

Solution Representation

Here, the solution is a 1D vector with N elements, where N implies the count of features in the original dataset. A field in a vector has the value of "1" or "0". Rate "1" indicates a similar feature as selected; otherwise, the rate "0" is retained.

Fitness Function

In this application, fitness function is applied to have an appropriate tradeoff between the count of features selected (minimum) and classification accuracy (maximum) obtained by using selected features. Fitness function to compute the solutions is calculated as follows:

$$\text{Fitness} = \propto \gamma_R(D) + \beta \frac{|R|}{|C|} \qquad (8.7)$$

where $\gamma_R(D)$ implies a classification error rate of the applied classier, $|R|$ denotes the cardinality of the selected subset, $|C|$ indicates the overall features present in a dataset, α and β are two parameters representing the importance of a subset length as well as classification supremacy. $[1, 0]$ and $\beta = (1 - \alpha)$ are taken from Ref. [25].

THE FRBC MODEL

Next to the FS process, the FRBC model is applied for classification purposes. Fuzzy classification models evolved from the rule-based approaches with massive benefits concerning performance and development. One of the major benefits of fuzzy classifiers is the interpretability of classification rules. Consider that $x = (x_1, x_2, \ldots, x_D) \in R^D$ is a D-dimensional feature space as well as $C = \{c_1, c_2, \ldots, c_m\}$ defines the collection of class labels. Following this, the classification issues are limited to define the class labels and a label signifies a feature vector of an object that has to be categorized. A fuzzy classification is provided using production rules as presented using Figure 8.5.

R_i: IF $s_1 \wedge x_1 = A_{1i}$ AND $s_2 \wedge x_2 = A_{2i}$ AND...AND $s_D \wedge x_D = A_{Di}$, THEN class = c_i, $i = 1, \ldots, R$, where A_{ki} implies a fuzzy term that classifies the k-th feature in the i-th fuzzy

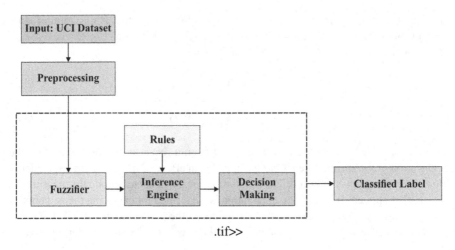

.tif>>

FIGURE 8.5 Fuzzy rule-based classification.

rule $(k = 1, \ldots, D)$, R means the value of fuzzy rules, and $S = (s_1, s_2, \ldots, s_D)$ denotes the binary feature vector while $s_k \wedge x_k$ represents the existence of $(s_k = 1)$ or inexistence $(s_k = 0)$ of a feature in a classification method.

From the applied dataset $\{(x_p; c_p), p = 1, 2, \ldots, Z\}$, a class label is demonstrated as given in the following:

$$\text{class} = c_t, t = \arg \max_{j=1,2,\ldots,m} \beta_j, m\beta j \tag{8.8}$$

$$\beta_j(xp) = \sum_{\substack{R_i \\ \text{class}_i = c_j}} \Pi_{k=1}^{D} \mu_{A_{ki}}(x_{pk}) \tag{8.9}$$

$\mu_{A_{ki}}(x_{pk})$ refers to the symmetric membership function (MF) for a fuzzy term A_{ki} at the point x_{pk}. Therefore, the value of the classifier is illustrated as a ratio among the number of accurately allocated class labels and the overall number of objects are categorized:

$$E(\Theta, S) = \frac{\sum_{p=1}^{Z} \begin{cases} 1, & \text{if } c_p = \arg_{j=1,2,\ldots m} \max f_j(x_p; \Theta, S) \\ 0, & \text{otherwise} \end{cases}}{Z}, \tag{8.10}$$

where $f(x_p; \theta, S)$ indicates the result of a fuzzy classifier with parameters θ and features S at a point x_p.

In order to develop a fuzzy classification model, two problems, namely fuzzy rule base generation and FS, have to be resolved. Initially, these problems are solved by emitting fuzzy rule base relied on higher values of a class, whereas the second problem is recovered using the optimization scheme. The fuzzy rule base generation model produces an initial rule base for a fuzzy classification with a single rule of a class. Therefore, rules are developed on the basis of extreme values in a training instances $T_r = \{(x_p; c_p), p = 1, 2, ..., Z\}$. Develop the given assumptions like m refers to the count of classes; D shows the count of features. A pseudo code of fuzzy rule base generation is illustrated in Algorithm 1.

Algorithm 1 Fuzzy Rrule Bbase Ggeneration Aalgorithm.

1: Input: m, T_r.
2: Output: fuzzy rule base R_i (where $i = 1, 2 ..., m$).
3: begin
4: for $i \leftarrow 1$ to m do
5:       for $k \leftarrow 1$ to D do
6:             Explore a left border of MF $\mu_{A_{ki}}(x_k)$:
7:             $a \leftarrow \min_{(p=1,2,...,Z) \wedge (c_p = i)} x_{pk};$
8: Explore a right border of MF $\mu_{A_{ki}}(x_k)$:
9:             $c \leftarrow \min_{(p=1,2,...,Z) \wedge (c_p = i)} x_{pk};$
10: Estimate a center of MF $\mu_{A_{ki}}(x_k)$:
11:         $b \leftarrow a + (c - a)/2;$
12: Develop symmetric triangular MF with borders a and c, as well as b for fuzzy A_{ki};
13: end
14: Develop rule Ri with $\mu_{A_{ki}}(x_k)$ MF ($k = 1, 2, ..., D$) and generates $c_k \leftarrow k;;$
15: end
16: end

EXPERIMENTAL RESULTS ANALYSIS

The performance of the proposed models is validated against three benchmark datasets namely Cleveland, Statlog, and Wisconsin dataset. The measures used to examine the diagnosis results are accuracy, sensitivity, specificity, F-score, and Matthews correlation coefficient (MCC). A comprehensive comparative results analysis is carried out with the existing models such as firefly (FF), PSO, grey wolf optimization (GWO), dragonfly algorithm, and F-DA models [25].

TABLE 8.1

Performance of the Proposed Model and Existing Models for the Cleveland Dataset

Measures	FF	PSO	GWO	DA	F-DA	WOA-FRBC
Accuracy	78.95	79.14	78.95	78.75	84.44	86.34
Sensitivity	37.21	39.54	37.21	34.88	51.16	60.26
Specificity	80.74	80.84	80.74	80.63	87.96	89.27
F-Score	12.70	13.49	12.70	11.90	38.59	40.20
MCC	08.91	10.12	08.91	07.70	31.55	40.23

RESULTS ANALYSIS ON THE CLEVELAND DATASET

Table 8.1 presents the performance of the WOA-FRBC model with existing techniques on the applied Cleveland dataset. The resultant values show that the WOA-FRBC model has achieved better results than all the other models.

For instance, on analyzing the results in terms of accuracy, the WOA-FRBC model has resulted in a higher accuracy of 86.34%, whereas the compared methods FF, PSO, GWO, DA, and F-DA models achieved lower accuracies of 78.95%, 79.14%, 78.95%, 78.75%, and 84.44%, respectively. In addition, on examining the results by means of sensitivity, the WOA-FRBC model has resulted in a higher sensitivity of 60.26%, while the compared models FF, PSO, GWO, DA, and F-DA models have resulted in least sensitivity values of 37.21%, 39.54%, 37.21%, 34.88%, and 51.16%, respectively. Along with that, on investigating the results in terms of specificity, the WOA-FRBC approach has led to a maximum specificity of 89.27% and the traditional schemes FF, PSO, GWO, DA, and F-DA models have exhibited minimum specificity values of 80.74%, 80.84%, 80.74%, 80.63%, and 87.96%, respectively. In line with this, on defining the results in terms of F-score, the WOA-FRBC model has provided a considerable F-score of 40.20%, while the compared technologies FF, PSO, GWO, DA, and F-DA models achieved lower F-scores of 12.7%, 13.49%, 12.7%, 11.9%, and 38.59%, respectively. Simultaneously, on analyzing the results by means of MCC, the WOA-FRBC model has resulted in a higher MCC of 40.23%, whereas the alternative methods FF, PSO, GWO, DA, and F-DA models achieved lower MCC values of 8.91%, 10.12%, 8.91%, 7.7%, and 31.55%, respectively.

RESULTS ANALYSIS ON THE STATLOG DATASET

Table 8.2 examines the function of the WOA-FRBC method with previous approaches on the given Statlog dataset. The final measures have implied that the WOA-FRBC model has achieved better results than all the alternate approaches. For instance, on analyzing the results in terms of accuracy, the WOA-FRBC model has implemented a maximum accuracy of 92.84%, whereas the compared technologies FF, PSO, GWO, DA, and F-DA models achieved lower accuracy values of 86.32%, 85.93%, 86.12%, 85.35%, and 86.5%, respectively. Additionally, on predicting the results in terms of sensitivity, the WOA-FRBC model has resulted in a higher sensitivity of 93.19%,

TABLE 8.2

Performance of the Proposed Model and Existing Models for the Statlog Dataset

Measures	FF	PSO	GWO	DA	F-DA	WOA-FRBC
Accuracy	86.32	85.93	86.12	85.35	86.50	92.84
Sensitivity	90.11	87.91	89.01	84.61	91.20	93.19
Specificity	85.95	85.74	85.85	85.43	86.05	90.56
F-Score	53.42	52.12	52.77	50.16	54.07	62.42
MCC	52.96	51.29	52.12	48.77	53.80	61.49

while the compared methods FF, PSO, GWO, DA, and F-DA models achieved lower sensitivity values of 90.11%, 87.91%, 89.01%, 84.61%, and 91.2%, respectively. Besides, on examining the results in terms of specificity, the WOA-FRBC model has resulted in a higher specificity of 90.56%, whereas the other methods FF, PSO, GWO, DA, and F-DA models achieved minimal specificities of 85.95%, 85.74%, 85.85%, 85.43%, and 86.05%, respectively.

Concurrently, on analyzing the results in terms of *F*-score, the WOA-FRBC model has resulted in a maximum *F*-score of 62.42%, whereas the compared methods FF, PSO, GWO, DA, and F-DA models achieved lower *F*-scores of 53.42%, 52.12%, 52.77%, 50.16%, and 54.07%, respectively. Eventually, on predicting the results in terms of MCC, the WOA-FRBC model has provided a maximal higher MCC of 61.49%, whereas the compared methods FF, PSO, GWO, DA, and F-DA models achieved lower MCC values of 52.96%, 51.29%, 52.12%, 48.77%, and 53.8%, respectively.

RESULTS ANALYSIS ON THE WISCONSIN DATASET

Table 8.3 predicts the function of the WOA-FRBC model with classical approaches on the applied Wisconsin dataset. The final values show that the WOA-FRBC model has achieved better results than all the other models. For sample, on analyzing the results in terms of accuracy, the WOA-FRBC model has provided supreme accuracy of 97.09%, whereas the compared methods such as FF, PSO, GWO, DA, and F-DA

TABLE 8.3

Performance of the Proposed Model and Existing Models for the Wisconsin Dataset

Measures	FF	PSO	GWO	DA	F-DA	WOA-FRBC
Accuracy	65.16	64.97	65.16	64.97	95.59	97.09
Sensitivity	8.62	8.04	8.62	8.04	100.00	100.00
Specificity	76.46	76.34	76.46	76.34	94.71	96.90
F-Score	7.61	7.10	7.61	7.10	88.32	92.78
MCC	−13.63	−14.26	−13.63	−14.26	86.55	91.05

models have achieved lower accuracy values of 65.16%, 64.97%, 65.16%, 64.97%, and 95.59%, respectively.

Moreover, on investigating the results with respect to sensitivity, the WOA-FRBC model has resulted in a higher sensitivity of 100%, whereas the compared methods such as FF, PSO, GWO, DA, and F-DA models resulted in limited sensitivity values of 8.62%, 8.04%, 8.62%, 8.04%, and 100%, respectively. Furthermore, on analyzing the results by means of specificity, the WOA-FRBC model has resulted in a higher specificity of 96.9%, whereas the compared methods FF, PSO, GWO, DA, and F-DA methodologies achieved lower specificities of 76.46%, 76.34%, 76.46%, 76.34%, and 94.71%, respectively. In the same way, on analyzing the results in terms of F-scores, the WOA-FRBC scheme has resulted in a higher F-score of 92.78%, whereas the compared approaches FF, PSO, GWO, DA, and F-DA models achieved minimum F-scores of 7.61%, 7.1%, 7.61%, 7.1%, and 88.32%, respectively. At the same time, on analyzing the results in terms of MCC, the WOA-FRBC framework has a projected superior MCC of 91.05%, whereas the compared schemes FF, PSO, GWO, DA, and F-DA models achieved lower MCC values of −13.63%, −14.26%, −13.63%, −14.26%, and 86.55%, respectively.

From the above-mentioned tables and figures, it is evident that the WOA-FRBC model has achieved an effective outcome over all the other methods. The experimental outcomes show that the WOA-FRBC model shows better diagnostic outcomes than the earlier techniques. The WOA-FRBC model achieves effective results owing to the automated rule generation of the FRBC model and optimal subset selection by WOA.

CONCLUSION

This chapter has developed an intelligent robot in the disease discovery process using the WOA-FRBC model. The WOA-FRBC model involves three distinct stages: preprocessing, FS, and classification. The input medical data are initially preprocessed by the robots to enhance the quality of the dataset. Then, the WOA-FS algorithm gets executed to extract an optimal feature subset. Following this, the FRBC technique is employed to identify the existence of the disease and determine the class label. The experimental outcomes show that the WOA-FRBC model has shown better diagnostic outcomes than the earlier techniques. The WOA-FRBC model achieves effective results owing to the automated rule generation of the FRBC model and optimal subset selection by WOA. As a part of future scope, the robots can be deployed in the real-time hospital environment to assist the physicians.

REFERENCES

1. Lu H, Li Y, Chen M, Kim H, Serikawa S. Brain intelligence: go beyond artificial intelligence. *Mobile Netw Appl* 2018;23(2):368–75.
2. Zhang N, Ding S, Zhang J, Xue Y. An overview on restricted Boltzmann machines. *Neurocomputing* 2018;275:1186–99.
3. Zhang J, Ding S, Zhang N, Shi Z. Incremental extreme learning machine based on deep feature embedded. *Int J Mach Learn Cybern* 2016;7(1):111–20.

4. Pustokhina IV, Pustokhin DA, Gupta D, Khanna A, Shankar K, Nguyen GN. An effective training scheme for deep neural network in edge computing enabled Internet of Medical Things (IoMT) systems. *IEEE Access* 2020;8(1):107112–23.

5. Lakshmanaprabu SK, Mohanty SN, Shankar K, Arunkumar N, Ramirez G. Optimal deep learning model for classification of lung cancer on CT images. *Future Gen Comput Syst* 2019;92:374–82.

6. Raj RJ, Shobana SJ, Pustokhina IV, Pustokhin DA, Gupta D, Shankar K. Optimal feature selection based medical image classification using deep learning model in Internet of Medical Things. *IEEE Access* 2020;8(1):58006–17.

7. Elhoseny M, Bian GB, Lakshmanaprabu SK, Shankar K, Singh AK, Wu W. Effective features to classify ovarian cancer data in Internet of Medical Things. *Comput Netw* 2019;159:147–56.

8. Shankar K, Sait AR, Gupta D, Lakshmanaprabu SK, Khanna A, Pandey HM. Automated detection and classification of fundus diabetic retinopathy images using synergic deep learning model. *Pattern Recogn Lett* 2020;133:210–16.

9. Sikkandar MY, Alrasheadi BA, Prakash NB, Hemalakshmi GR, Mohanarathinam A, Shankar K. Deep learning based an automated skin lesion segmentation and intelligent classification model. *J Ambient Intell Humaniz Comput* 2020:1–11. doi: 10.1007/s12652-020-02537-3.

10. Shi K, Wang J, Zhong S, Zhang X, Liu Y, Cheng J. New reliable nonuniform sampling control for uncertain chaotic neural networks under Markov switching topologies. *Appl Math Comput* 2019;347:169–93.

11. Xu X, Lu H, Song J, Yang Y, Shen HT, Li X. Ternary adversarial networks with self-supervision for zero-shot cross-modal retrieval. *IEEE Trans Cybern* 2019;50:2400–13.

12. Mohan S, Thirumalai C, Srivastava G. Effective heart disease prediction using hybrid machine learning techniques. *IEEE Access* 2019;7:81542–54.

13. Loey M, Smarandache F, M Khalifa NE. Within the lack of chest covid-19 x-ray dataset: anovel detection model based on gan and deep transfer learning. *Symmetry (Basel)* 2020;12(4):651.

14. Zhou T, Canu S, Ruan S. An automatic COVID-19 CT segmentation based on U-Net with attention mechanism. arXiv preprint arXiv:200406673, 2020.

15. Ghoshal B, Tucker A. Estimating uncertainty and interpretability in deep learning for coronavirus (COVID-19) detection. arXiv preprint arXiv:200310769, 2020.

16. Nilashi M, bin Ibrahim O, Ahmadi H, Shahmoradi L. An analytical method for diseases prediction using machine learning techniques. *Comput Chem Eng* 2017;106:212–23.

17. Zhang C, Zhu L, Xu C, Lu R. PPDP: an efficient and privacy-preserving disease prediction scheme in cloud-based e-healthcare system. *Future Generat Comput Syst* 2018;79:16–25.

18. Chen X, Niu Y-W, Wang G-H, Yan G-Y. Hamda: hybrid approach for mirna-disease association prediction. *J Biomed Inform* 2017;76:50–8.

19. Parisot S, Ktena SI, Ferrante E, Lee M, Guerrero R, Glocker B, Rueckert D. Disease prediction using graph convolutional networks: application to autism spectrum disorder and alzheimers disease. *Med Image Anal* 2018;48:117–30.

20. Weng C-H, Huang TC-K, Han R-P. Disease prediction with different types of neural network classifiers. *Telemat Informat* 2016;33(2):277–92.

21. Kumar PM, Lokesh S, Varatharajan R, Babu GC, Parthasarathy P. Cloud and IoT based disease prediction and diagnosis system for healthcare using fuzzy neural classifier. *Future Generat Comput Syst* 2018;86:527–34.

22. Luo J, Ding P, Liang C, Chen X. Semi-supervised prediction of human mirna-disease association based on graph regularization framework in heterogeneous networks. *Neurocomputing* 2018;294:29–38.

23. Sengupta S, Das AK. Particle swarm optimization based incremental classifier design for rice disease prediction. *Comput Electron Agric* 2017;140:443–51.
24. Mafarja M, Mirjalili S. Whale optimization approaches for wrapper feature selection. *Appl Soft Comput* 2018;62:441–53.
25. Koppu S, Maddikunta PKR, Srivastava G. Deep learning disease prediction model for WWuse with intelligent robots. *Comput Electr Eng* 2020;87:106765.

9 Biomedical Healthcare Robot Movement Control Using an EEG-Based Brain–Computer Interface with an Optimized Kernel Extreme Learning Machine

S. Stephe and T. Jayasankar
Anna University

CONTENTS

INTRODUCTION

Basically, mammals communicate by the electrical and chemical signals generated in them. Electrophysiology is assumed as a subclass of physiology used in observing electrical activities related to body parts. The electrophysiological data are recorded by fixing the electrodes wherever required. For this purpose, massive approaches were applied for tracking the electrical activity and electrophysiological data in different organs like the heart, brain, eyes, cells, stomach, and so on [1–3]. Electroencephalography (EEG) is a well-known electrophysiological model applied for observing the electrical function of the brain by locating the electrodes on the head scalp [4]. EEG is mainly applied to save the differences in voltage caused due to the flow of ionic power in the internal portion of the brain's neurons. Hence, EEG signals are in the form of waves named brainwaves that represent the neural oscillations generated by neurons.

A brain–computer interface (BCI) is one of the well-known systems used for identifying the communication between the brain and machines. For effective disease diagnosis, the brain signals are recorded, distributed, and generates required rules for a connected device [5]. Hence, the BCI method is applied in various domains like integrity and authentication, academics, neuromarketing, and broadcasting, games, and many other clinical domains like cognitive neuroscience, brain-relied elimination and diagnosis of health issues, rehabilitation, and restoration [6–8]. The task of BCI depends upon the frequent implementation of best strategies such as signal acquisition, preprocessing, feature extraction, classification, conversion, as well as providing feedback to the operator [9], as illustrated in Figure 9.1.

The EEG-related BC robot is defined as a robot that applies EEG-relied BCI to receive managing commands from a user. As an inclusion, EEG-based BC mobile

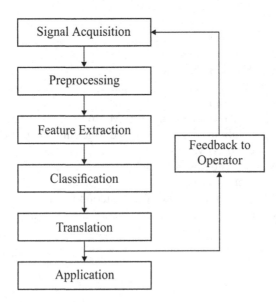

FIGURE 9.1 Process in the BCI model.

robots are supportive for old-age people and handicapped users with destructive neu-romuscular infections like amyotrophic lateral sclerosis (ALS), multiple sclerosis (MS), and so on. This module is classified into two aspects, namely BC manipula-tors and BC mobile robots. Likewise, assistive mobile robots are divided into two classes based on their performance mode [11]. The basic class is composed of assis-tive mobile robots that are operated by direct BCI control [10]. This kind of robot is managed by commands received from users and sends them to BCI modules, with no guidance by robot intelligence units. For this sake, it is cheaper and complicated to make accurate motion control. Besides, the entire function of the BC mobile robots relies on the BCI function, which results in insufficient speed of response as well as accuracy. Moreover, the requirement for the frequent generation of the motor con-trolling commands by users is tiring.

The primary instances of a robot are projected in a study [11], where the left- and right-turning actions of a robotic wheelchair are managed directly by the motion commands converted from the user brain signals. Likewise, in another study [12], a BC mobile robot was made to move front, left, and back and right directions with the help of a BCI that relied on motor imagery. In addition, in Ref. [13], the wheelchair motion control is operated by a BCI, which is composed of alpha brainwaves. In par-ticular, collection of icons corresponds to prior commands as they appear on a screen and the user is able to decide the required command by closing the eyes as soon as the icon is displayed in a display unit. Secondly, the class is composed of assistive mobile robots operated under distributed control. Following this, the robots of this class are operated by integrating the BCI system with smart controllers, like an independent navigation system. Besides, the deployment is costlier with maximum processing complexity.

A general example of distributed control in assistive mobile robots was given in the study of Mandel et al. [14]. In this study, the steady-state visually evoked poten-tials (SSVEP) BCI system is applied with the capability of sending the commands to change the robotic wheelchair in four various directions whereas the independent navigation system implements delivered commands. In line with this, in Ref. [15], with the help of P300 BCI, an operator applies previous locations for selecting a required position and forwards the selection to an independent navigation system where the robotic wheelchair is guided to move in the defined destination. Along with that, in Ref. [16], shared control has been applied. In particular, the integrated application of P300 BCI with an autonomous navigation system has been presented for computing motion control of a robotic wheelchair in an unseen platform. In addition, the user is capable of moving the wheelchair in the desired direction by concentrating on two relative icons at the previous visual display. In Ref. [17], three mental operations, which consider the right and left-hand movements as well as the word generation that are initialized with an identical random letter. Finally, the system used in this model communicates with the user under the application of the PDA screen that is applicable in guiding a robotic wheelchair in known as well as in unknown platforms.

This chapter introduces a new robot movement control technique using electroencephalography (EEG)-based BCI with an optimized kernel extreme learning machine (KELM), called BCI-OKELM. The BCI-OKELM model comprises different stages of signal acquisition, preprocessing, feature extraction, and classification. Primarily, signal preprocessing is performed by removing the noise using filtering techniques and min-max normalization is used. In addition, the OKELM model is applied as a feature extractor followed by the inbuilt softmax (SM) layer for the classification process. For tuning the hyperparameters of the KELM model, an improved particle swarm optimization (IPSO) algorithm is employed. To investigate the betterment of the BCI-OKELM model, diverse simulation experiments are performed and the results are compared with several models.

This chapter is organized as follows. "The Proposed BCI-OKELM Model" section introduces the BCI-OKELM model, the "Experimental Evaluation" section presents the simulation analysis, and the "Conclusion" section concludes the study.

THE PROPOSED BCI-OKELM MODEL

The working of the presented BCI-OKELM model is explained here. As depicted, the input signals are initially captured and preprocessed using two stages, namely filtering for noise removal and min-max for normalization processes. Next to preprocessing, OKELM-based feature extraction and SM-based classification processes are performed. Besides, the IPSO algorithm is applied to identify the optimum values of the hyperparameters that exist in the KELM model.

DATA ACQUISITION USING BCI AND ROBOTS

Here, the BCI device applied tends to enhance the alpha brainwaves at the time of the experimental process carried out in Open BCI Ganglion [18]. Hence, a robot applied for implementing the experimental strategy is a crawler robot developed on Dagu Rover 5 Chassis. A Raspberry Pi (model 3 B+) is facilitated as the central processing unit (CPU) for a robot. Communication between a robotic vehicle and a system can be accomplished by TCP or IP socket connection. Once the classifier has determined fixed action, a command is forwarded to the robot. Therefore, serial communication is introduced among the Raspberry Pi and the Arduino UNO microcontroller. After receiving the command, it depends upon the microcontroller to apply the L298N H-Bridge driver mechanism to balance the motors of a robot.

DATA PREPROCESSING

In EEG-BCIs, signal acquisition is carried out with the help of electrodes placed in the scalp of the user. Preprocessing is a step performed for eliminating the noise and outliers present in the signal and few filtering approaches are also employed to eliminate the interruptions caused by endogenous sources like eye movements, muscles, and heart disease, and exogenous sources like power-line combination as well as an impedance mismatch. In general, preprocessing is carried out by the application of low-pass, high-pass, band-pass, or notch filtering. Hence, a second-order IIR notch filter with a quality factor Q is employed for eliminating the frequency (50 Hz). Min–max normalization was employed for feature scaling from the rank of [0,1], which is then saved in a dataset.

KELM-BASED CLASSIFICATION

In recent times, the ELM mechanism with robust learning speed as well as optimal generalization function has gained maximum interest from developers [19]. In this approach, the basic parameters of the hidden layer are not tuned and most of the non-linear piecewise continuous functions are employed as hidden neurons. Hence, for N random distinct instances $\{(x_i, \ t_i) | \ x_i \in R^n, t_i \in R^m, i = 1,..., N\}$, the final expressions in ELM with L hidden neurons are

$$f_L(x) = \sum_{i=1}^{L} \beta_i h_i(x) = h(x)\beta \tag{9.1}$$

where $\beta = [\beta_1, \beta_2, \beta_L]$ means a vector of output weights among a hidden layer of L neurons and resultant neuron and $h(x) = [h_1(x), \ h_2(x),...,h_L(x)]$ implies the resultant vector of the hidden layer by means of input x that maps the data from input to ELM feature space.

In order to reduce the training error and to enhance the generalization function of NN, the training error as well as final weights have to be reduced simultaneously as defined in the following:

$$\text{Minimize: } \|H\beta - T\|, \|\beta\| \tag{9.2}$$

The least-squares solution of (9.2) relies on KKT conditions as defined below:

$$\beta = H^T \left(\frac{1}{C} + HH^T\right)^{-1} T \tag{9.3}$$

where H means a hidden layer output matrix, C defines a regulation coefficient, and T signifies the desired result matrix.

Next, the final expression of the ELM learning model is as follows:

$$f(x) = h(x)H^T \left(\frac{1}{C} + HH^T\right)^{-1} T \tag{9.4}$$

If feature mapping $h(x)$ is referred to as unknown and the kernel matrix of ELM depends upon Mercer's conditions, then

$$M = HH^T: m_{ij} = h(x_i)h(x_j) = k(x_i, x_j) \tag{9.5}$$

Hence, the last function $f(x)$ of a KELM is defined as follows:

$$f(x) = [k(x,x_1),...,k(x,x_N)] \left(\frac{1}{C} + M\right)^{-1} T \tag{9.6}$$

where $M = HH^T$ and $k(x, y)$ refers to the kernel function of the hidden neurons from single hidden layer feed-forward neural networks (SLFN).

162   Robotic Technologies

Massive kinds of kernel functions were developed to meet the Mercer condition; some of them are the linear kernel, polynomial kernel, Gaussian kernel, and exponential kernel. The structure of KELM is shown in Figure 9.2. Here, three types of kernel functions (KF) are used for simulation and performance validation for selected KF as given below.

(1) Gaussian kernel:

$$k(x,y) = \exp(-a \| x - y \|) \tag{9.7}$$

(2) hyperbolic tangent (sigmoid) kernel:

$$k(x,y) = \tan h(bx^T y + c) \tag{9.8}$$

(3) wavelet kernel:

$$k(x,y) = \cos\left(d\frac{\| x - y \|}{e}\right) \exp\left(-\frac{\| x - y \|^2}{f}\right) \tag{9.9}$$

where Gaussian KF is considered as general and local KF, whereas tangent KF is considered as common global nuclear function, correspondingly. Moreover, complex wavelet KF is applied for testing the developed models. From the above KF,

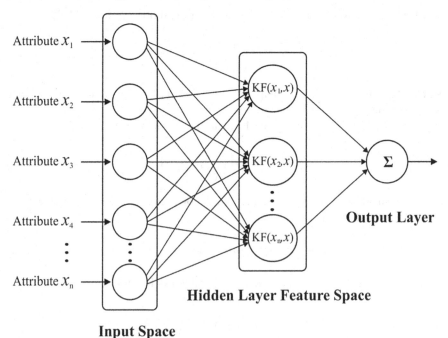

FIGURE 9.2 The structure of the KELM model.

the tunable parameters a, b, c, e, and f are highly essential, which have to be tuned effectively on the basis of the resolved problem. When the comparison task is performed, hidden layer feature mapping is not considered in KELM. Additionally, the KELM learning model gains the same generalization function, which is compared with the classical ELM and it is robust when compared with a support vector machine (SVM).

IPSO-BASED PARAMETER TUNING OF THE KELM MODEL

To tune the hyperparameters of the KELM model, the IPSO algorithm is employed. Recently, various optimization models have been developed to solve complex problems. The PSO method is a population-based stochastic optimization approach developed by Dr. Eberhart and Dr. Kennedy in 1995, where the social behaviors of bird gathering and fish schooling were studied. These structures are initiated by the population of random simulations and explore the optimal generation. PSO lacks deployment operators like mutation and crossover. In PSO, possible solutions named as elements fly with complicated space by using recent optimal solutions. Because of the maximum efficiency, PSO is applied under various domains and even the real-time channels have adopted, especially in multimodal problems. Hence, it is referred to as an effective model used to overcome the clustering issues. Here, the PSO approach is applied for resolving the software-defined problems significantly and the flowchart of the PSO algorithm is shown in Figure 9.3. However, PSO is considered an inferior model of local exploring convergence, especially in composite multi-peak search issues. Thus, in contrast to the above-defined issues, traditional PSO is extended by expanding the inertial weight and maintaining particles from trapped local optima, which has applied the extended PSO method for fitness purposes. Finally, additional CH and dispatch nodes are selected from a protocol. It is operated on five stages, as defined in the following.

Initializing the Optimization Problem and Algorithm Parameters

Develop the finite count of elements. Here, the particle size is implied as M; each element e is composed of a speed vector $s_e = [s_{e1}, s_{e2}, ..., s_{ed}]$ and a position vector $q_e = [q_{e1}, q_{e2}, ..., q_{ed}]$ and has been applied for pointing the recent state, in which i denotes a positive integer in a swarm and d refers to the dimensions of a problem.

Calculating the Fitness Values

The elements found in d-dimensional hyperspace manipulated the fitness values of an element based on (9.5) and (9.8). Using the search principle, an element monitors the personal optimal (pbest) solution $P_e = [p_{e1}, p_{e2}, ..., p_{ed}]$ and the global optimal (gbest) solution $P_g = [p_{g1}, p_{g2}, ..., p_{gd}]$ accomplished with various elements in a swarm.

Updating Velocity and Position Vectors

Each phase affects the speed of an element at gbest and pbest locations. The speed of an element is defined as follows:

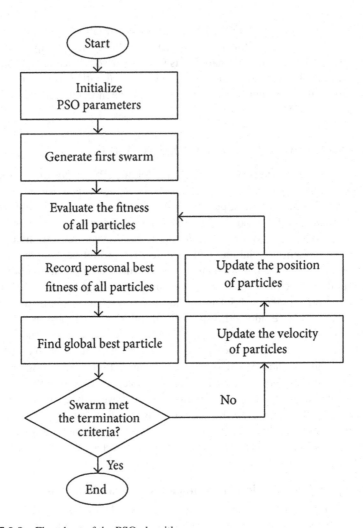

FIGURE 9.3 Flowchart of the PSO algorithm.

$$s_{ef}^{z+1} = w s_{ef}^z + cr\left(p_{ef}^z - q_{ef}^z\right) + cr\left(p_{gf}^z - q_{gf}^z\right) \tag{9.10}$$

with the location of elements described as follows:

$$q_{ef}^{z+1} = q_{ef}^z + s_{ef}^{z+1} \tag{9.11}$$

where s_{ef} is the fth dimension of the eth element's speed, which is ensured by a nearby range of $\left[s_{mn}, s_{mx}\right]$ in order to terminate the explosion of elements. The information of q_{ef}, p_{ef} and p_{gf} depends upon the s_{ef}. Coefficients r_1 and r_2 are two randomly developed values from [0,1] for the dth dimension. c_1 and c_2 indicate two acceleration variables that are allocated as 2.0. Factor w means the inertial weight that contributes to managing previous efficacy of an element that balances among global search (maximum inertial weight) as well as local search (minimum inertial weight).

Changing the Inertial Weight

In order to maintain a distance from declining as local optimum, the extended version of PSO has been applied to change the inertial weight based on Eq. (9.13), which prevents elements from being trapped in local optima:

$$w = \left(w_{mx} - w_{mn}\right) \times \frac{\text{Iteration}_{mx} - \text{Iteration}_e}{\text{Iteration}_{mx}} + w_{mn} \qquad (9.12)$$

where w_{mx} and w_{mn} refer to the maximum and minimum inertial weights, respectively. Iteration$_{mx}$ denotes the maximum values of considerable iterations, and Iteration$_e$ implies the present iteration.

Going to Step 3 Until the Termination Criterion Is Met

The projected best solutions are selected until reaching the stopping criterion. It is assumed to be a resolution for optimization issues.

EXPERIMENTAL EVALUATION

This section examines the performance of the presented BCI-OKELM model under different perspectives. Table 9.1 presents the binary values associated with the movement of the robots. For instance, the binary sequence of '1010' directs the robot to move in the forward direction. Similarly, the binary sequence of '0101' directs the robot to move in the reverse direction. Along with that, the binary sequence of '1100' directs the robot to move in the left direction. At last, the binary sequence of '0011' directs the robot to move in the right direction.

Figure 9.4 shows the accuracy graph generated by the BCI-OKELM model under varying numbers of epochs. The figure shows that the BCI-OKELM model has resulted in higher training and validation accuracy. These values tend to increase with an increase in the number of epochs. Comparatively, the validation accuracy has seemed to be high compared to the training accuracy. The BCI-OKELM model has achieved a minimum training and validation accuracies of 0.6 and 0.56 at the

TABLE 9.1

Binary Values Associated with the Movement of the Robots

Sequence	Movements
1010	Forward
0101	Reverse
1100	Left
0011	Right

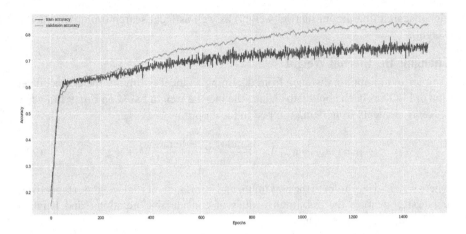

FIGURE 9.4 Accuracy analysis of the BCI-OKELM model.

beginning of the epoch count and reached a maximum of 0.85 and 0.75 at the training and validation accuracies on the higher epoch count of 1,400.

Figure 9.5 shows the loss graph produced by the BCI-OKELM model under a variable number of epochs. The figure shows that the BCI-OKELM model has attained reduced loss under training and validation loss. These values tend to decrease with an increase in the number of epochs. Relatively, the validation loss has seemed to be lower compared to the training loss. The BCI-OKELM model has attained higher training and validation accuracies of 0.18 and 0.85 at the beginning of the epoch count and reached a maximum of 0.3 and 0.25 at the training and validation accuracies on the higher epoch count of 1,400.

A comprehensive comparative results analysis of the BCI-OKELM model is carried out in terms of sensitivity and specificity with the ANN, ANFIS, MLP, LR, and XGBoost models. The comparative outcome is provided in Table 9.2.

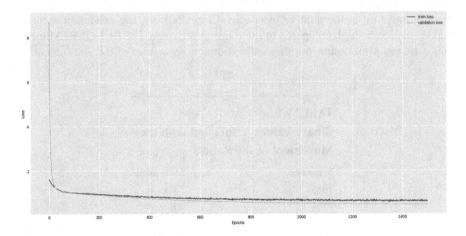

FIGURE 9.5 Loss graph analysis of the BCI-OKELM model.

TABLE 9.2

Result Analysis of Various Classification Methods

Methods	Precision	Accuracy
BCI-OKELM	76.85	85.70
ANN	69.41	69.36
ANFIS	74.59	72.75
MLP	64.59	67.09
LR	70.08	70.11
XGBoost	75.00	75.13

On determining the classification performance of the BCI-OKELM model, the MLP model has resulted in a minimum sensitivity of 68.45%. Besides, the ANN model has achieved a slightly higher performance with a sensitivity of 68.73%. Upon continuation, the LR model has obtained a moderate classification outcome with the sensitivity of 69.48%, whereas the ANFIS model has obtained a moderate accuracy of 70.61%. In line with this, a competitive sensitivity of 74% has been accomplished by the XGBoost model.

However, the projected BCI-OKELM model showed effective classification with an increased sensitivity of 81.36%. On computing the classification function of the BCI-OKELM method, the XGBoost approach has resulted in a least specificity of 61%. Besides, the MLP model has achieved considerable performance with a specificity of 63.91%. Upon continuation, the ANN model has attained reasonable classification results with the specificity of 67.97%, whereas the LR model has obtained a better accuracy of 73.03%. Likewise, a competitive specificity of 74% has been achieved by the ANFIS scheme. Hence, the proposed BCI-OKELM model has implied effective classification with the maximum specificity of 87.24%.

Table 9.3 presents the precision and accuracy analysis of diverse models. On evaluating the classification function of the BCI-OKELM model, the MLP model has

TABLE 9.3

Precision and Accuracy Analysis of Various Classification Methods

Methods	Precision	Accuracy
BCI-OKELM	76.85	85.70
ANN	69.41	69.36
ANFIS	74.59	72.75
MLP	64.59	67.09
LR	70.08	70.11
XGBoost	75.00	75.13

resulted in a lower precision of 64.59%. Following this, the ANN model has achieved an acceptable function with a precision of 69.41%. Upon continuation, the LR model has obtained a slightly better classification outcome with the precision of 70.08%, whereas the ANFIS model has obtained a reasonable accuracy of 74.59%. In line with this, a competitive precision of 75% has been obtained by the XGBoost method. However, the developed BCI-OKELM approach has implied efficient classification with the enhanced precision of 76.85%.

On estimating the classification performance of the BCI-OKELM scheme, the MLP scheme has attained a minimal accuracy of 67.09%. Besides, the ANN model has achieved a moderate performance with an accuracy of 69.36%. Upon continuation, the LR model has obtained a better classification result with an accuracy of 70.11% while the ANFIS model has obtained a moderate accuracy of 72.75%. In line with this, a competing accuracy of 75.13% has been achieved by the XGBoost scheme. Therefore, the presented BCI-OKELM approach has depicted proficient classification with the maximum accuracy of 85.70%.

From the analysis of the above-mentioned results, it is evident that the BCI-OKELM model shows superior performance with the sensitivity, specificity, precision, and accuracy of 81.36%, 87.24%, 76.85%, and 85.70%, respectively.

CONCLUSION

This chapter has introduced a new robot movement control technique using the EEG-based BCI with optimized KELM, called BCI-OKELM. The BCI-OKELM model comprises different stages of signal acquisition, preprocessing, feature extraction, and classification. The presented model controls the movement of the robots based on the blinking of the operator's eye through the EEG-based BCI, which makes use of alpha brain waveforms. The input signals are initially captured and preprocessed using two stages namely filtering for noise removal and min-max for normalization processes. Next to preprocessing, OKELM-based feature extraction and SM-based classification processes are performed. Besides, the IPSO algorithm is applied to identify the optimum values of the hyperparameters that exist in the KELM model. A set of experiments were performed to highlight the better results of the BCI-OKELM model. The resultant values showed proficient performance with the maximum sensitivity, specificity, precision, and accuracy of 81.36%, 87.24%, 76.85%, and 85.70%, respectively. In the future, advance deep learning (DL) models can be utilized instead of KELM for improving the classification outcome.

REFERENCES

1. Dixon, A.M.; Allstot, E.G.; Gangopadhyay, D.; Allstot, D.J. Compressed sensing system considerations for ECG and EMG wireless biosensors. *IEEE Trans. Biomed. Circuits Syst.* 2012, 6, 156–166.
2. Perdiz, J.; Pires, G.; Nunes, U.J. Emotional state detection based on EMG and EOGbiosignals: A short survey. In *Proceedings of the 2017 IEEE 5th Portuguese Meeting on Bioengineering (ENBENG)*, Coimbra, Portugal, 16–18 February 2017; pp. 1–4.

3. Valais, I.; Koulouras, G.; Fountos, G.; Michail, C.; Kandris, D.; Athinaios, S. Design and construction of a prototype ECG simulator. *EJST* 2014, 9, 11–18.
4. Wolpaw, J.R.; Birbaumer, N.; McFarland, D.J.; Pfurtscheller, G.; Vaughan, T.M. Brain–computer interfaces for communication and control. *Clin. Neurophysiol.* 2002, 113, 767–791.
5. Abdulkader, S.N.; Atia, A.; Mostafa, M.S.M. Brain computer interfacing: Applications and challenges. *Egypt. Inform. J.* 2015, 16, 213–230.
6. Katona, J.; Kovari, A. A Brain–computer interface project applied in computer engineering. *IEEE Trans. Educ.* 2016, 59, 319–326.
7. Katona, J.; Kovari, A. The evaluation of BCI and PEBL-based attention tests. *Acta Polytech. Hung.* 2018, 15, 225–249.
8. Katona, J.; Kovari, A. Examining the learning efficiency by a brain-computer interface system. *Acta Polytech. Hung.* 2018, 15, 251–280.
9. Nicolas-Alonso, L.F.; Gomez-Gil, J. Brain computer interfaces, a review. *Sensors* 2012, 12, 1211–1279.
10. Bi, L.; Fan, X.A.; Liu, Y. EEG-based brain-controlled mobile robots: A survey. *IEEE Trans. Hum. Mach. Syst.* 2013, 43, 161–176.
11. Tanaka, K.; Matsunaga, K.; Wang, H.O. Electroencephalogram based control of an electric wheelchair. *IEEE Trans. Robot.* 2005, 21, 762–766.
12. Choi, K.; Cichocki, A. Control of a wheelchair by motor imagery in real time. In *Proceedings of the International Conference on Intelligent Data Engineering and Automated Learning*, Daejeon, Korea, 2–5 November 2008; Springer: Berlin, Germany, 2008; pp. 330–337.
13. Ferreira, A.; Silva, R.L.; Celeste, W.C.; Bastos, T.F.; Filho, M.S. Human–machine interface based on muscular and brain signals applied to a robotic wheelchair. *J. Phys. Conf. Ser.* 2007, 90, 1–8.
14. Mandel, C.; Luth, T.; Laue, T.; Röfer, T.; Graser, A.; Krieg-Bruckner, B. Navigating a smart wheelchair with a brain–computer interface interpreting steady-state visual evoked potentials. In *Proceedings of the 2009 IEEE/RSJ International Conference on Intelligent Robots and Systems*, St. Louis, MO, USA, 10–15 October 2009; pp. 1118–1125.
15. Rebsamen, B.; Burdet, E.; Guan, C.; Zhang, H.; Teo, C.L.; Zeng, Q.; Ang, M.; Laugier, C. A brain controlled wheelchair based on P300 and path guidance. In *Proceedings of the 1st IEEE/RAS-EMBS International Conference on Biomedical Robotics and Biomechatronics*, Pisa, Italy, 20–22 February 2006; pp. 1001–1006.
16. Iturrate, I.M.; Antelis, J.; Kubler, A.; Minguez, J. A noninvasive brain-actuated wheelchair based on a P300 neurophysiological protocol and automated navigation. *IEEE Trans. Robot.* 2009, 25, 614–627.
17. Benevides, A.B.; Bastos, T.F.; Filho, M.S. Proposal of brain–computer interface architecture to command a robotic wheelchair. In *Proceedings of the IEEE International Symposium in Industrial Electronics*, Gdansk, Poland, 27–30 June 2011; pp. 2249–2254.
18. Korovesis, N., Kandris, D., Koulouras, G. and Alexandridis, A. Robot motion control via an EEG-based brain–computer interface by using neural networks and alpha brainwaves. *Electronics* 2019, 8(12), 1387.
19. Li, B., Rong, X. and Li, Y. An improved kernel based extreme learning machine for robot execution failures. *Sci. World J.*, 2014, 2014, 906546.

Index

Note: Page numbers in *italics* and **bold** refer to figures and tables.

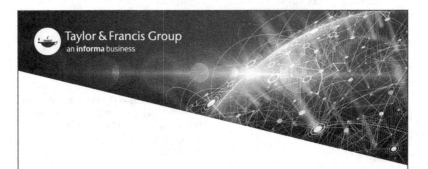

Printed in the United States
by Baker & Taylor Publisher Services